**PRAISE FOR**

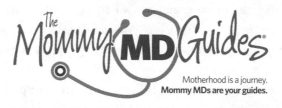

Motherhood is a journey.
**Mommy MDs are your guides.**

It is fascinating to find the real experiences of physician moms interposed with solid data about healthy pregnancy and delivery. *The Mommy MD Guide to Pregnancy and Birth* is an enjoyable and enlightening book that will "hold hands" with women through their pregnancies.

> —*Joanna M. Cain, MD, Chace/Joukowsky Professor and chair, assistant dean of women's health at the Warren Alpert Medical School of Brown University, and obstetrician and gynecologist-in-chief at Women & Infants Hospital, both in Providence, RI*

*The Mommy MD Guide to Your Baby's First Year* is fun, easy to read, and informative. I love that the advice from physicians is practical and based on experience, in addition to medical expertise.

Since it is a series of vignettes, it's easy to read and pick up in between other activities, which is ideal for busy people like me and new moms.

> —*Jennifer Arnold, MD, a neonatologist and the medical director of the Pediatric Simulation Center at Texas Children's Hospital and an assistant professor at Baylor College of Medicine, both in Houston, and the star of TLC's* The Little Couple

*The Mommy MD Guide to the Toddler Years* is a great testament to the fact that no two kids or parents are exactly alike. I am always looking for new ideas for entertaining, disciplining, teaching, and loving on my kids because what worked with my first child doesn't always work with the other five! I love that this book accepts, appreciates, and addresses the fact that there isn't just one answer to any question or concern parents have with their children. For me, the more suggestions I can get, the better!

—*Casey Jones, a mom of a 9-year-old daughter and 4-year-old quintuplets and costar of* Quints by Surprise, *in Austin, TX*

I found a quiet corner in the living room and flipped open *The Mommy MD Guide to Pregnancy and Birth*, about a topic I last experienced 10 years ago. The more I read, the more I kept thinking to myself, "I wish this book had been *around* 10 years ago." I would have devoured every word if I'd read it 20 years ago, as I plodded through my very first experience with the baffling world of pregnancy. This book really is different from every other pregnancy book I've read.

*The Mommy MD Guide to Pregnancy and Birth* has advice from 60 doctors who are moms. Aside from the great medical advice, I was drawn to the anecdotal feeling of this book. As I read, I felt like I was sitting in the living room with these women as they shared their personal stories. I'm a person who loves to hear a good birth story, and I was really drawn to the personal nature of the advice. Instead of feeling like it was coming from a textbook, the advice feels like it's coming from a girlfriend who's just navigated the road herself. But it went beyond "just" a girlfriend's guide, because it was a girlfriend's guide times 60.

I highly recommend *The Mommy MD Guide to Pregnancy and Birth*. I have a feeling many dads wouldn't mind reading it either since it's not long chapters of information, but short snippets of advice, gathered in a very logical way.

I enjoyed the website that's hosted by the authors and look forward to the series this team is working on, covering the other stages of parenting, from newborn sleep issues to elementary school struggles. It's a great idea that was truly done right.

—*Judy Berna, a mom of four and writer for GeekMom.com*

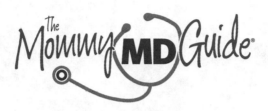

# The Mommy MD Guide®

## to
# Getting
# Your Baby
## to
# Sleep

*The*
Mommy **MD** Guide®
to
# Getting
# Your Baby
to
# Sleep

**More Than 400 Tips That 38 Doctors Use
to Get Their Kids to Sleep — So You Can Too!**

By Rallie McAllister, MD, MPH
and Jennifer Bright Reich

© 2016 by Momosa Publishing LLC

Printed in the United States of America

Illustrations by Carrie Wendel

Book design by Leanne Coppola

Library of Congress control number available upon request.
ISBN 978–0–9844804–8–7

2  4  6  8  10  9  7  5  3  1  paperback

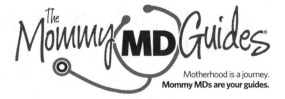

Motherhood is a journey.
**Mommy MDs are your guides.**

MommyMDGuides.com

*To my sisters, Gayle and Nancy*
*—RM*

*To my mom—I miss you every hour of every day.*
*—JBR*

# Contents

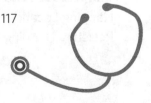

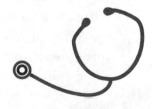

# Acknowledgments

The books in the Mommy MD Guides series are proof positive that if we dream big, work hard, and believe in ourselves, we can accomplish anything we feel passionate about. If we're lucky enough to have the help and support of friends and family while we're at it, the process is a whole lot easier, and a lot more fun.

I feel incredibly blessed to have Jennifer as a friend, coauthor, and business partner. Although it's roughly 600 miles from my desk to hers, she's as close to me as a sister. Jennifer and I are both passionate about helping moms carry out one of the most important jobs in the world—raising healthy, happy children. We couldn't do this without the help of our awesome team at the Mommy MD Guides or the incredible physicians who generously shared the stories of their lives. I'm grateful to each of them.

I'm also grateful to my family—Robin, Oakley, Gatlin, Chad, Lindsey, Bella, Cam, and Anna—and very thankful for all the love and laughter we share.

—*Rallie McAllister, MD, MPH*

❧

First and foremost, thank you so very much to Rallie. You make every day at Momosa Publishing a great day. Your energy, optimism, wisdom, ideas, and strength always amaze me. I will always be grateful to you!

Thank you to the 150+ Mommy MD Guides who shared their stories and experiences with us for our books and MommyMDGuides.com. The best part of my job is meeting and talking with smart, funny, fascinating, and kind people like you! Thank you for sharing your tips and wisdom with us.

Many thanks also to the Mommy MD Guides team. I'm so fortunate to work with such a talented group: editor Amy Kovalski, consultant Jennifer Goldsmith Cerra, advisor Mary Lengle, writer Marie Suszynski, proofreader Ashley Kuhn, designer Leanne Coppola, researcher Jennifer Kushnier, layout designer Susan Eugster, illustrator Carrie Wendel, indexer Nanette Ben-dyna, and printing manager Karen Kircher.

I am very grateful to Drew Frantzen, our logo designer, who helped to establish the very tone and style of our brand.

Thank you to my mentors and friends who have shared their wisdom and advice: Susan Berg, Elly Phillips, Chris Krogermeier, Anne Egan, Joey Green, Tim Foster, Colleen Krcelich, Andrew K. Gonsalves, and Buddy Lesavoy.

Most of all, thank you to my family—Tyler and Austin Reich and John R. Bright, Mary L. Bright, Robyn Swatsburg, and Judy Beck—for all of your support, encouragement, and love and for making my life so rich, rewarding—and fun.

—*Jennifer Bright Reich*

# Introduction

I've looked forward to writing this book for 10 years! Sleep was elusive for the first five years after my boys were born. The catalyst to create the Mommy MD Guides book series was a conversation I had 10 years ago with my sons' pediatrician about how she got her own children to sleep. She shared how she got her four little ones to sleep, and her tips worked for me, too.

To create this book, we spoke with 38 Mommy MD Guides—doctors who are also mothers. These doctors shared their stories, tips, and tricks about how they got their own babies and kids to sleep. Some of them were blessed with "good sleepers," while others struggled with "not-so-good sleepers" or faced challenges only at particular points in their children's lives.

These smart, funny, fascinating women opened their hearts and lives to us. They shared their challenges with bedtime, naps, illnesses, and crying. They also talked with us about celebrating when their babies slept through the night, date nights with their partners, and transitioning their toddlers to beds.

The more than 400 tips and stories in this book are presented in the Mommy MD Guides' own words, and each tip is clearly attributed to the doctor who *lived* it. Most of these stories contain kernels of advice. This is what doctors who were also new mothers did to help their babies sleep better. Other stories in this book are just that—true stories. The implied advice is: I made it through this pesky problem, and you can too!

Even though this book is filled with advice from a select group—all Mommy MD Guides—you'll find that they hold vastly differing opinions. We've presented many different viewpoints—but not with the intent to confuse or to offer conflicting advice. Instead, these diverse voices are presented so that you can choose what's best for you as you navigate your own parenting journey.

As you read this book, keep in mind that every child, mother, and family is different. Babies—and moms!—face different challenges with sleep. Things change and improve at different speeds for everyone. Not all progress is the same, and not all progress is linear. You might have some ups and downs. You might experience some plateaus—even some setbacks.

Welcome to the Mommy MD Guides! Best wishes for your health and happiness, great sleep, and sweet dreams!

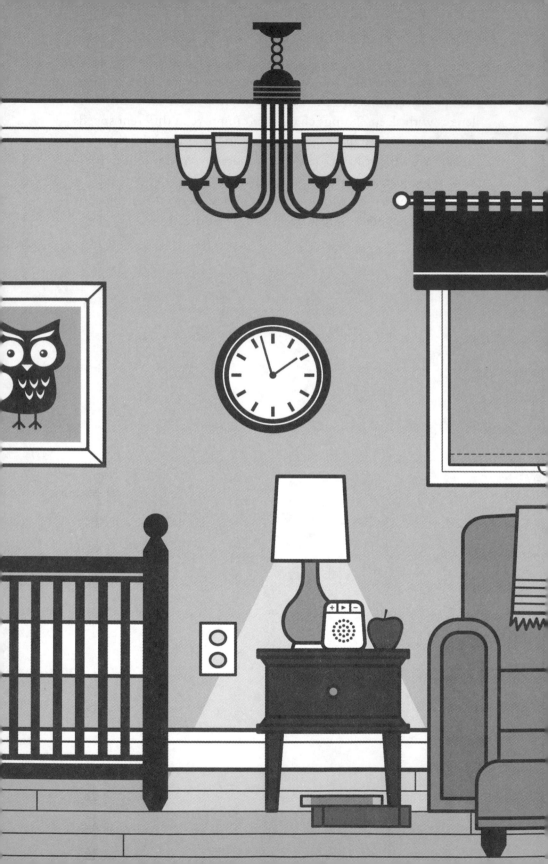

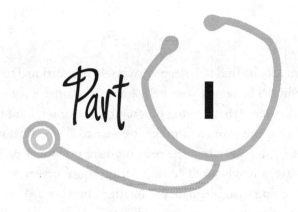

# NEWBORNS: BIRTH TO 1 MONTH

# Chapter 1

## Sleeping in the Hospital

Many moms-to-be find that sleep is inversely proportional to the size of their bellies. The bigger your belly gets, the harder it is to sleep.

It makes sense that if being pregnant is making it hard to sleep, then not being pregnant will make it easier to sleep. That's perfect logic—until you realize that the reason you're no longer pregnant is you that have a newborn. The only thing more inversely proportional to sleeping than pregnancy is having a newborn.

For those nights when you and your baby are in the hospital, your chances of sleeping are better. There's a cadre of highly trained labor and delivery nurses right outside your hospital door! The nurses will offer you advice, they'll do everything they can to help make you comfortable, and they'll even take your baby to the hospital nursery or nurse's station if you'd like.

We urge you to take them up on any and all of these options. Think about it: You'll probably never find more experienced people to look after your little one than those nurses!

### JUSTIFICATION FOR A CELEBRATION

Congratulations and best wishes on the birth of your new baby! The best is yet to come!

> **People who say they sleep like a baby usually don't have one.**
>
> —*Leo J. Burke, psychologist*

## Rooming-In with Your Baby

You've spent a long 40 weeks waiting, thinking, hoping, and dreaming about your new baby. It's a safe bet you want to spend every waking second looking into that perfect little face. Choosing rooming–in seems like a no–brainer.

Fortunately, experts support this. The Baby-Friendly Hospital Initiative, a global program of the World Health Organization (WHO) and the United Nations Children's Fund (UNICEF), developed 10 Steps to Successful Breastfeeding. Not surprisingly, one of those 10 steps is rooming–in, allowing mothers and infants to remain together 24 hours a day.

A review from the *Cochrane Library*, a collection of health databases, finds some evidence that rooming–in supports breast-feeding, at least in the short term. The review showed that babies who roomed in with their mothers were more likely to be breast-feeding when they were four days old than babies who slept in the hospital nursery. Surprisingly, studies show new moms get more sleep with their babies in the room.

Just because your baby is in the room doesn't mean you have to be alone every second! Don't hesitate to ask the nurses for help. They are experts in brand new babies, and you'll likely find them eager and willing to help.

&#x221D;

When my babies were born, by C-section, they were placed right to my breast. Even though I was half out of it, I was very glad they did that. It's instinct for the baby to go to the breast.

For the few nights my babies and I were in the hospital, they roomed in with me. Now it's usually policy to do so. I found it was helpful to have my babies with me to establish good nursing and also for me to begin to learn my babies' cues when they were hungry, tired, etc.

—*Eva Mayer, MD, a mom of a 12-year-old daughter and an 11-year-old son, an associate professor of pediatrics at Temple University, and a pediatrician with St. Luke's Hospital Coopersburg Pediatrics, in Pennsylvania*

In the hospital, for all three births, I wanted to keep my babies in the room with me so I could cherish those early moments, and also have easy access to nurse as needed. I loved creating a little cocoon for just the two of us, and although I was exhausted, I didn't want to miss a minute of those first hours and days of life.

—*Rebecca Kempton, MD, a mom of eight- and six-year-old sons and a three-year-old-daughter and an infant and toddler sleep specialist, in Chicago, IL*

When I was in the hospital for the birth of my new baby, we roomed in. My baby slept well. She woke every two to three hours to eat. Usually in the hospital, if your baby rooms in with you, the baby will sleep in a hospital bassinet, on her back, swaddled.

—*Aline T. Tanios Keyrouz, MD, a mom of 13- and 7-year-old and 9-month-old daughters and an 11-year-son and an assistant professor of pediatrics at St. Louis University, in Missouri*

When my babies were born, hospital nurseries were rare. If new moms needed a few hours without their babies to rest, the nurses would wheel the babies out to the central nurses' area.

This worked out fine for me. My babies roomed in with me, and I nursed them on demand. But I did ask the nurses to take them out to the nurses' area for a few hours at night so I could sleep.

My babies and I didn't stay in the hospital long, though. I prefer sleeping in my own bed and being in my own home!

—*Marcela Dominguez, MD, a mom of a 13-year-old daughter and an 11-year-old son who has a private family medicine and wellness practice in Southern California, whose concierge medicine services are provided by Signature MD*

When my babies were born, I roomed in with all four of them in the hospital. I really wanted to use those first two days to establish nursing.

As awesome as the breastfeeding policies might be at a hospital, a lot of factors impact breastfeeding if they bring your baby to you or give him a bottle. I know from doing newborn nursery rotations during my residency that if you tell the nurses that you want the baby brought to you, they try really hard to do that. But a nurse might misremember, a new nurse might not check first, they might not want your baby to

## Mommy MD Guides–Recommended Product
### Saving Mothers Safe Birth Kits

"Because no woman should die giving life."

That's the simple, dramatic tagline for Saving Mothers, a non-profit organization dedicated to eradicating preventable maternal deaths in developing countries. Founded and run by medical professionals, Saving Mothers recognizes that the vast majority of these deaths occur due to lack of access to quality healthcare and or even basic sanitary medical supplies. Shocked and saddened by the scope of this problem—more than 343,000 die during childbirth every year—founders Dr. Taraneh Shirazian and Dr. Nichole Young-Lin resolved to mobilize whatever resources they could to effect change in this area.

One of their simplest and most effective interventions is the Saving Mothers Safe Birth Kit. At a cost of only $10, each kit contains everything that even the most minimally skilled birth attendants need to ensure safe deliveries outside of the hospital setting: soap to cleanse the birth mothers' perineum, a shower curtain to provide a clean surface for delivery, rubber gloves, and a razor blade to cut the umbilical cord. These ordinary items are essential to preventing the spread of infection during delivery.

You can help save a new mother's life for less than it would cost to treat you and your BFF to Starbucks. As you hold this book in your hands—and probably your baby in your arms—think back to when you packed your own "kit" to prepare for your hospital stay. Wouldn't it be nice to provide a safe birth kit to a pregnant mother a world away and enable her to survive to see her baby grow up? To learn more, visit **WWW.SAVINGMOTHERS.ORG/SAFE _ BIRTH _ KITS**.

get upset, or it might be a change of shift and too chaotic, and they might give your baby a bottle anyway. Also, it might be protocol that if a baby gets too cold, they give an ounce of formula. Often, they give babies bottles with the best of intentions.

A breastfeeding baby having a bottle isn't tragic. But I wanted my babies to have the best chance of getting the hang of nursing.

Another reason why I wanted to breastfeed as much as possible in the hospital was that I wanted us to learn how to do it in the hospital where support was available if I had questions. I wanted them to teach me how to fish, not *hand* me a fish.

*—Deborah Gilboa, MD, a mom of 14-, 12-, 10-, and 8-year-old sons, a family physician with Squirrel Hill Health Center, in Pittsburgh, PA, and a parenting speaker whose advice is found at AskDoctorG.com*

In the hospital, my babies and I slept in the same room. I had twins and a C-section. I was exhausted. In hindsight, I wish I had taken advantage of having the girls sleep in the nursery, to get some much needed rest. But having them in the room with me was a wonderful bonding time!

*—Sonal R. Patel, MD, a mom of four-year-old twin daughters and a physician who specializes in pediatric/adult allergy and immunology with Adventist Health Physicians Network, in Los Angeles, CA*

## Baby Sleeping in the Hospital Nursery

The best laid plans of mice—and *moms*—do sometimes go awry! Yes, you might have had a 3$\frac{1}{2}$-page double-spaced birth plan, witnessed by your husband, and signed by your midwife. But if you just endured 21 hours of labor, 5$\frac{1}{2}$ hours of pushing, and a C-section, you're probably exhausted. Your body, your mind, and your soul need sleep.

You have a lifetime to spend with your baby. Take the few precious hours the hospital will give you, and send your baby to the nursery so you can rest!

## BABY SLEEP PRO TIP: Target Sleep Times

Like so many things in life, our needs for sleep change as we grow and develop. Here's a basic guide to our changing sleep needs.

| AGE | NIGHT SLEEP (HOURS) | DAY SLEEP (HOURS) | TOTAL (HOURS) |
|---|---|---|---|
| Newborn-2 months | 8-10* | 7-9 (3-5 naps) | 17-20 |
| 2-4 months | 9-11* | 4-5 (3-4 naps) | 14-16 |
| 4-6 months | 10-12* | 4-5 (2-3 naps) | 14-15 |
| 6-9 months | 11-12* | 3-4 (2 naps) | 14 |
| 9-12 months | 11-12 | 2-3 (2 naps) | 14 |
| 12-18 months | 11-12 | 2-3 (1-2 naps) | 13-14 |
| 18 months- 2 years | 11-12 | 2 (1 nap) | 13-14 |
| 2-3 years | 11-13 | 1-2 (1 nap) | 12-14 |
| 3-5 years | 11-13 | 0-1 | 11-13 |
| 5-7 years | 10-12 | 0 | 10-12 |

*not necessarily continuous sleep, may include wakings for feedings

—*Rebecca Kempton, MD*

When I had my kids, the nurses took my baby to the nursery. New moms really didn't have much of a choice. That was back when fathers were just starting to be allowed in the delivery room.

When my first grandchild was born, my daughter's husband was in the room with my daughter the entire time they were in the hospital. This gave my daughter a chance to bond with her baby that I didn't have, and it also gave me a chance to help her learn to hold her baby properly and change his diapers while she was still in the hospital.

I remember when I went home with my first daughter, I laid her on the bed and thought, *Now what do I do?*

—*Kathryn Boling, MD, a mom of two grown daughters, a grandmom of two, and a family medicine physician with Mercy Medical Center, in Baltimore, MD*

Even if your baby goes to the hospital nursery to sleep, try to breastfeed. Breastfeeding has been associated with a 60 percent reduction in SIDS deaths, especially in babies who were exclusively breastfed. One review study showed that the longer the baby was breastfed, the greater the protective effect against SIDS. This connection may be linked to breast milk's protective effects against infections.

—*Rebecca Kempton, MD*

～

When my babies were born, I planned to have them room in with me. My oldest roomed in. When my youngest baby was born, I woke up in the hospital after a nap, and he was gone! They had checked his bilirubin level, and it was high, and so they took him to the nursery— without telling me.

Of course I wanted them to treat him, but I felt they should have let me know first! I had a nice talk with the staff. I explained I needed to know when my baby was going to be checked.

When the baby isn't with you, a nurse might give him a pacifier

## Getting Sleep Yourself in the Hospital

After just giving birth, there's no better "me" time when you're not tending to your baby than blissful sleep. You need it now more than ever, but how do you get restful shut-eye in a bustling hospital?

Physical activity during the day helps, so start by taking walks around the maternity ward in the morning and afternoon. Also avoid caffeine after 12 pm and eat dinner three hours before you plan to turn in. Avoid disruptions by telling friends you're not taking visitors during the late evening hours. At bedtime, create a sleep environment in your room by turning off the television and other electronic devices, lowering the shades, turning off the lights, and donning an eye mask and ear plugs if you need to. You can also try relaxation techniques, such as deep breathing or meditation and listen to soothing sounds on a smartphone app.

or even formula, which you might not want if you're trying to nurse. I
went to the nursery every hour and a half to make sure my baby was
getting my milk.

—*Sharon Boyce, MD, a mom of seven- and five-year-old sons
and a family physician with Oaklawn Medical Group, in Albion
and Bellevue, MI*

When I was in the hospital after giving birth, I ran into a friend from
medical school. We both just had our babies, on the same day! This
was her second child and my first.

As my friend was doing her walk around the floors as required
by the nurses, she peeked into my hospital room and asked, "Can I
give you some advice?"

I welcomed *any* advice from a mother who was also a doctor.

My friend said, "Don't keep that baby in the room with you. Give
him to the nurses during the day and at night except when you need
to feed him."

I was surprised. I was a new mother who had been trying to get
pregnant for so long, and I had already lost a child to miscarriage. All I
wanted to do was keep this baby in my sight and in my arms. But I took
my friend's advice to heart and I followed it. Consequently, I felt I was
better able to heal and get caught up on sleep (outside of feeding the
baby). I was able to take care of myself and get my strength back. I was
recovering from a C-section, which is major abdominal surgery.

I was so grateful for my friend's advice that I passed it on at all of my prenatal visits as a pediatrician. I followed the same advice with my second child.

My friend also advised me to use the maximum number of days allowed by my insurance to stay in the hospital to recover. My insurance plan allowed me four days, and I took all four days. It was a blessing.

I think these new rules of eliminating the hospital nursery and having moms spend more time with their babies the first few days after birth are not doing right by the moms. Moms need this time to rest and recover. They will have forever to be with and take care of their babies. They need those first few days to take care of *themselves*. Do right by yourself and your baby and give yourself time to rest and recuperate in the few days after the birth of your little one.

—*Nilong Parikh Vyas, MD, MPH, a mom of seven- and five-year-old sons and the founder and owner of Sleepless in NOLA sleep consulting, in New Orleans, LA*

## RALLIE'S TIP

*After nine months of pregnancy, I was so happy to finally have each of my babies out of my belly and in my arms! Each was a perfect, tiny miracle, and I could hardly take my eyes or my hands off them.*

*Immediately after my sons were born, I remember being completely overcome by the intense love that I felt for my newborn babies, and also by a ferocious sense of mother-bear protectiveness. There was no way I was letting those babies out of my sight for a minute longer than necessary.*

*When my oldest son was born, rooming-in wasn't an option. The nurses whisked my baby away to the nursery according to schedule.*

*By the time my two younger sons were born years later, rooming-in was the norm, and I was allowed to keep them with me in my hospital room. I had a far better experience when I kept my babies with me. I felt that we bonded more completely, breastfeeding went more smoothly, and I was happier in the post-partum period.*

*As long as mom and baby are healthy, I think it's important for them to be together, with skin-to-skin contact, as much as possible in the hours and days after birth. Early, close contact is critical for mother-child bonding.*

# Chapter 2
## Deciding Where the Baby Sleeps

When you and your baby first come home from the hospital, you might not have a whole lot of control over when your baby sleeps. Babies from birth up to four months old don't have sleep patterns yet. Their sleep isn't even related to daylight and nighttime cycles. Most new babies sleep for two to four hours, multiple times a day. Be patient! Your baby's sleep patterns won't begin to emerge until after she's six weeks old.

What you do have control over is where your baby sleeps. You might all sleep best if your baby sleeps in her nursery. Or perhaps you'll sleep better if she sleeps in your room in a crib or bassinet. Or maybe the best solution for your family is a co-sleeper. It all comes down to what works best for your family.

### JUSTIFICATION FOR A CELEBRATION
The first night you and your baby sleep in your home is definitely a reason to celebrate.

> **Sometimes the smallest things take up the most room in your heart.**
> —*Winnie the Pooh*

## Baby Sleeping in the Nursery

The American dream might be a home to call your own, but the American *mom's* dream is a perfectly decorated nursery with a beautiful baby sleeping in it.

Nursery safety is, of course, critical. Your baby's crib must be her safe haven. When choosing a crib, don't put your baby in a used crib with drop-down sides. In 2011 the U.S. Consumer Product Safety Commission banned traditional drop-side cribs that were manufactured before June 2011. Why? The moveable sides could detach and entrap, suffocate, or strangle a baby.

Here's to a beautiful nursery and beautiful dreams for your baby—and for you.

❧

Being a pediatrician, I knew not to start any bad habits like nursing my baby to sleep. From his first day at home, my baby slept in his crib, in the dark.

—*Michelle Davis-Dash, MD, a mom of a five-year-old son and a pediatrician, in Baltimore, MD*

❧

I'm married to another physician, and we used to both take call 24/7 from home. To prevent our baby hearing the phones ring, he started sleeping in his own room when he was only two months old. It was winter, so we made it warm and dark, and he loved it!

—*Larissa Guerrero, MD, a mom of a three-year-old son and family practice physician with Healthrow Ob/Gyn in Orlando, FL*

❧

I absolutely under no circumstances *ever* allowed my newborn in bed with me. It's incredibly dangerous. There is no way to ever "make it safe." I've seen the consequences of this in the emergency department, and it can be fatal.

—*Lisa M. Campanella-Coppo, MD, a mom of a six-year-old daughter and an emergency department physician at Summit Medical Group, in Livingston, NJ*

My husband and I had our babies sleep in their bedrooms as much as possible so that they would learn bedrooms are for sleeping. We played with them in common areas to reinforce this.

—*Rebecca Jeanmonod, MD, a mom of 12- and 8-year-old daughters and 11- and 8-year-old sons and a professor of emergency medicine and the associate residency program director for the emergency medicine residency at St. Luke's University Health Network, in Bethlehem, PA*

~⌒~

We had a bassinet in our bedroom. But my baby didn't sleep there for long because every little sound she made woke *me* up. Because I slept so poorly with her near me, we had her sleep in her crib in her room, which was next to ours. My daughter slept well from early on, two to four hours at a go.

—*Katja Rowell, MD, a mom of a 10-year-old daughter, a family practice physician, and the author of* Helping Your Child with Extreme Picky Eating and Love Me, Feed Me *at* TheFeedingDoctor.com, *in St. Paul, MN*

## Mommy MD Guides-Recommended Product

### Convertible Cribs

Most moms have to watch their dollars—and sense! That's why we love any product that does double duty. If you haven't already bought your baby's crib, consider a convertible one.

Many convertible cribs allow you to adjust the height of the mattress as your baby gets bigger and begins to sit and then stand. This is practical, and it's also important for safety.

Convertible cribs can usually be used for babies and toddlers up to 36 months. Then, you can simply and easily convert the crib into a toddler bed, daybed, or full-size bed. It's important to check before you buy if you need to purchase any conversion parts separately! For example, you might need to buy separate conversion rails.

Convertible cribs cost around $275. You can buy them in stores such as Target and online such as on **AMAZON.COM**.

After the first few months, when my babies were sleeping through the night, after their night nursing, my husband would take them back to their rooms. He would just put them in the crib and leave. It was like he was thinking, *I want my wife back now.*

*—Sharon Boyce, MD, a mom of seven- and five-year-old sons and a family physician with Oaklawn Medical Group, in Albion and Bellevue, MI*

Our kids never slept in our bed. They became so accustomed to sleeping in their rooms that they didn't even want to sleep in our bed.

One time when my husband was out of town, I told my kids we could have a slumber party in my room—watch movies, read books, and they could sleep there. They were excited, but when it was time for bed, my daughter announced she was going to her room to sleep!

When I asked why, my daughter said, "Because it's the most comfortable bed in the house!"

My son said, "I'm sleeping with Momma."

But my daughter said, "Oh no you don't! It wouldn't be fair. If I'm sleeping in *my* bed, you have to sleep in *your* bed!"

*—Lauren Hyman, MD, a mom of a 13-year-old daughter and an 11-year-old son and an ob-gyn at West Hills Hospital and Medical Center, in California*

## Baby Sleeping in Your Room

You've enjoyed the past 40 weeks—give or take a few—with your baby a *part* of you. It's probably unimaginable to think of her sleeping in a separate crib, in a separate room, down the hall. She might as well be in another state!

That's why many new moms choose to have their newborns sleep in their rooms. Some moms move the crib into their rooms; others have their babies sleep in bassinets. Moms have plenty of support for this. The American Academy of Pediatrics' official position is that the safest place for a baby to sleep is in her crib or bassinet in the parents' room, close by the bed.

This is also supported by good ol' fashioned common sense.

> **If people were meant to pop out of bed,
> we'd all sleep in toasters.**
>
> —*Author unknown, attributed to Jim Davis*

If your baby sleeps in your room, you'll hear her easier and get to her more quickly. This might just result in less crying on her part—and on yours.

❧

During my twins' first four months, they slept in a co-sleeper in our bedroom. This was convenient so that they could be nearby for feedings and diaper changes. When they were four months old, we moved them to a crib in their own room. They were small enough to share the same crib. They enjoyed being near each other, and this helped ease the transition.

*—Sonal R. Patel, MD, a mom of four-year-old twin daughters and a physician who specializes in pediatric/adult allergy and immunology with Adventist Health Physicians Network, in Los Angeles, CA*

❧

My babies' beds were in our bedroom for the first few weeks—just for convenience for breastfeeding during the night. Once night feeding was over, we moved their beds to their own room.

*—Ayala Laufer-Cahana, MD, a mom of 20- and 18-year-old sons and a 17-year-old daughter, a pediatrician, artist, entrepreneur, and founder of Herbal Water Inc. and DrAyala.com, in greater Philadelphia, PA*

❧

All three of my children slept in a bassinet or Pack 'n Play near our bed in our room for the first three months of life. I always felt more at ease knowing they were nearby and safe. This also helped with feeding during the night because we didn't have to travel as far to get them when it was time for them to nurse.

*—Sigrid Payne DaVeiga, MD, a mom of 10-year-old and 1-month-old sons and a 5-year-old daughter and a pediatric allergist with the Children's Hospital of Philadelphia, in Pennsylvania*

I brought my babies home from the hospital the day after they were born because I thought we'd all be happier at home. But I wanted to sleep in the same room with them at first. I wanted to be able to wake up and look at them! We put our newborns next to our bed.

After three or four days, we moved the babies into rooms of their own. It worked out wonderfully.

—*Elizabeth Berger, MD, a mom of two grown children, a child psychiatrist, and the author of* Raising Kids with Character, *in New York City*

For my babies' first few weeks, we had them sleep in a Pack 'n Play next to our bed. As the kids got older, we taught them that Mom and Dad's bedroom is our little sanctuary. When we ask them to leave, it's time to leave. Even if they have nightmares, they can come in and get consoled for a bit, but then it's time to go back to their rooms.

—*Antoinette Cheney, DO, a mom of a 12-year-old son and an 11-year-old daughter, and a family physician with Rocky Vista University College of Osteopathic Medicine, in Parker, CO*

My babies generally slept well, and we were fortunate not to have a lot of sleeping issues. The hardest part for me was how exhausted I was for the first six weeks when my babies slept in a bassinet in my room.

From the beginning, I was careful not to pick up my babies every time they made a noise. Babies are noisy sleepers! If they woke up before feeding time, I would wait for a few minutes to see if they would fall back to sleep. If the baby kept fussing, I would quietly press her hand next to her mouth so she could learn to pacify on her own.

When my babies were six weeks old, I moved them into cribs in their rooms.

—*Marcela Dominguez, MD, a mom of a 13-year-old daughter and an 11-year-old son who has a private family medicine and wellness practice in Southern California, whose concierge medicine services are provided by Signature MD*

There was never a question as to where the baby would sleep when he first came home.

When each of our boys came home as newborns, they slept in our room with us in their own separate space. We had a bassinet for them. Thinking back now, it wasn't approved for sleeping safely, but back then there were no Pack 'n Play systems. This worked out fine for us. Today, I would use an approved co-sleeper, such as a Pack 'n Play.

—*Leena S. Dev, MD, a mom of teenage boys and a general pediatrician, in Maryland*

Initially, when my babies first came home from the hospital, they slept in a basket by the bed to make breastfeeding easier those first weeks. After the first month or so, I moved my babies into a crib in my bedroom so I could still breastfeed easily during the night.

## Mommy MD Guides–Recommended Product
### Halo Bassinest Swivel Sleeper

The Halo Bassinest Swivel Sleeper is a co-sleeper and bassinet in one. Its base fits underneath your bed so you can pull the bassinet next to you at eye level as you sleep. The bassinet includes mesh walls that lower so it's easy to pick up your baby, especially if you're recovering from a Cesarean section. It also swivels 360 degrees so you're able to get out of bed easily. The bassinet is recommended for babies up to 20 pounds who aren't yet rolling over or pushing up.

The sleeper comes with a fitted sheet and fits beds that are 22 inches to 34 inches high. It comes in four models that run from $199.99 to $299.99. Additional features on the more expensive models include a soothing center that provides vibration for the baby, plays lullabies and soothing sounds, and has a nursing timer, nightlight, floor light, and storage caddy.

Visit **HALOBASSINEST.COM** for more information.

When my babies were around four or five months old and they were sleeping longer between feedings, I moved them—and the cribs—into their own rooms.

—*Kathryn Boling, MD, a mom of two grown daughters, a grandmom of two, and a family medicine physician with Mercy Medical Center, in Baltimore, MD*

Although my first baby co-slept with me, my other three babies slept in a bassinet and then advanced to a crib. Because of changing life situations and my medical career obligations, co-sleeping wasn't an option. I used a bassinet for the first three months or so. I always tried to keep my babies as close to me as possible, especially during the first three months when bonding is key.

When my babies began to gain motor strength, I moved them to a crib.

—*Hana R. Solomon, MD, a mom of four grown biological children, two grown "spiritually adopted" children, a grandmom of eight, a pediatrician, the president of BeWell Health, LLC, the inventor of Dr. Hana's Nasopure nose wash for children, and the author of* Clearing the Air One Nose at a Time: Caring for Your Personal Filter, *in Columbia, MO*

My babies never slept with us. We did have them in a bassinet in our room for about the first six weeks.

I breastfed each of my six children. I was "lazy," and I didn't want to get up in the middle of the night—every two hours—and have to trek all the way into another room to fetch the baby to nurse and then bring him back to bed. Having the baby in my room was easier.

It was even easier than that actually. My husband and I made a deal: Because he couldn't breastfeed, he was in charge of the fetch and carry. He didn't need to travel so far to fetch, and I didn't have to get out of bed in the middle of the night!

After six weeks, the nursing pattern stabilized and was more predictable, so it was easier to plan those nightly feedings. At that point, the baby was moved to a full-sized crib. We all slept better then!

*—Susan Besser, MD, a mom of six grown children, a grandmom of five, and a family physician at River Family Physicians, in Easton, MD*

## Co-Sleeping with Your Baby

Sometimes in life, you have to weigh what experts say, compare it with what experts *do*, and make the best decision for yourself and for your family. The question of co-sleeping is a perfect example of this.

The American Academy of Pediatrics (AAP) and the U.S. Consumer Product Safety Commission *both* urge parents not to have their babies sleep in the parents' bed, due to the risk of suffocation. But at the end of the (long, long) day, however, many exhausted moms resort to bed-sharing to get some much-needed sleep. According to Parents.com, 65 percent of moms have slept in bed with their infants, and 38 percent do so regularly.

Perhaps the best strategy is a compromise. The AAP okays using a co-sleeper, which is a bassinet that attaches securely to the

### Pampering Yourself with a Beautiful Bedroom

If you have put your focus solely on the baby's nursery and have neglected your bedroom, take time now to create a comfortable and pleasing room. It can help you sleep better and give you a calm place to retreat at the end of the day, making those peaceful hours after your baby drifts off to sleep extra soothing for you.

Start with a supportive mattress that's less than 10 years old, which ensures the quality you need for a good night's sleep, the National Sleep Foundation says. Add in good pillows and bedding, along with furniture that is comfortable and inviting. Keep the room free of clutter, papers, electronics, and work materials, and choose a wall color that you find to be soothing, such as blue or green, which are thought to bring on feelings of peace and calm.

side of the parents' bed. A co-sleeper makes it quick and easy to get to your baby, but because your baby isn't in the grown-up bed, she doesn't have the risk of suffocation. This will help you breathe easier too.

❧

Our firstborn slept in her crib in the nursery from the beginning. But as a first-time mom, I stayed up all night staring at the monitor to make sure she was still breathing.

So our second child slept in a co-sleeper in our room. I was a little more relaxed, and this still allowed me to check on him frequently. Plus, the nursery is down the hallway, so it was easier to have him right there for frequent feedings.

—*Jennifer Bacani McKenney, MD, a mom a five-year-old daughter and a three-year-old son and a family physician, in Fredonia, KS*

❧

When my kids were babies, they generally slept in their cribs in their own rooms. But if I was exhausted, they might have fallen asleep with me sometimes.

The American Academy of Pediatrics cautions about co-sleeping because studies show that adults and children do not get as high quality sleep, and it increases the risk of SIDS up until 12 months. However, I tell parents in certain instances it is helpful. Don't get angry with yourself if you are exhausted, your child is sick, etc, if you fall asleep with her. You must always follow SIDS guidelines. (See www.healthy-children.org.)

Don't make yourself nuts; do what works for your family. As long as a parent isn't very overweight, abusing substances, or a very heavy sleeper, it's natural to want to have your baby with you. One important caveat: Both parents have to be on the same page about this.

—*Eva Mayer, MD, a mom of a 12-year-old daughter and an 11-year-old son, an associate professor of pediatrics at Temple University, and a pediatrician with St. Luke's Hospital Coopersburg Pediatrics, in Pennsylvania*

When my younger daughter was born, we were living in Miami. The concept of the family bed is strong there, so we went with that. My baby would wake up, nurse or just cuddle, and go back to sleep.

I know family beds are frowned upon in many cultures, and some fear that you could roll on your child and injure her. Many parents complain that they can't get restful sleep this way. However, I found it much easier than getting up during the night to nurse. Getting the best night's sleep possible is important for everyone involved, especially when you're going to work in the morning.

—*Eva Ritvo, MD, a mom of two grown daughters, a psychiatrist, and a coauthor of* The Beauty Prescription, *in Miami Beach, FL*

I co-slept with my first baby. At the time, we were living in a one-room cabin with only a wood fire for heat and no running water! I needed my baby to sleep near my body to keep her warm.

Also, I believed because my baby was inside of me for nine months, it was only natural to have my baby skin to skin right next to me for the first few weeks. My baby felt secure, I felt secure, and this was best suited for us.

I wasn't worried about rolling over or suffocation because I felt confident in a mother's survival skills to keep a baby safe. Evolution supports this idea.

## ♥ Buy the Best Mattress

If your mattress or pillow is more than 9 or 10 years old, purchasing a new one could contribute to better sleep. Here are some mattress-choosing tips from the Better Sleep Council.

• Wear comfortable clothing and take off your jacket and shoes.

• Lie down in your normal sleeping position and make some turns too.

• If the bed's for two, try it together.

• If you have back pain, choose a supportive rather than a hard bed. Often a medium-firm bed is the best option.

> **Without enough sleep,
> we all become tall two-year-olds.**
> —*JoJo Jensen*, **Dirt Farmer Wisdom**, *2002*

As my other children arrived, life variables affected my choices. During my medical residency, working 110 hours per week, and breastfeeding 100 percent, I didn't have the luxury to co-sleep. Then my husband did the co-sleeping and bottle-feeding with breast milk for 12 months. I was in survival mode, and I caught sleep whenever I could.

    —*Hana R. Solomon, MD*

&#x223D;

Before my first baby was born, we had purchased an arm's-reach co-sleeper. This was so the baby could sleep next to me—but in his own space—so I could easily feed him through the night as needed.

However, after the first few days of being home, I quickly realized that my son was a very noisy sleeper. He made so many noises in the middle of the night that would wake me up and make me stare at him for long periods of time wondering if he was still breathing or uncomfortable or needing to eat. I wondered, *Why is he making these noises. Does he need something?*

I realized after multiple wakings that my baby didn't need anything at all. He was just a noisy sleeper. That's when we made the decision to move him to a crib in his room. His crib was next to the wall that separated our bedrooms. We left the bedroom doors open, and we had a monitor on our nightstand. This helped because we still felt close to him and knew when he was truly hungry. I could hear him cry and go to him, but I wasn't being woken by every little noise and movement. We all slept better from that point forward because I wasn't attending to every single movement and whimper on his part, and he was able to work on getting himself back to sleep if needed.

This really helped me, and I think it is great advice for new parents. We all want to be very close to our babies, but we need to give them "space" to sleep, and the parents need their "space" to sleep as well. Your baby will let you know if something is wrong—if he is having trouble falling back to sleep, or if he's hungry, wet, uncomfortable, or in pain.

—*Nilong Parikh Vyas, MD, MPH, a mom of seven- and five-year-old sons and the founder and owner of Sleepless in NOLA sleep consulting, in New Orleans, LA*

When we brought our babies home, I co-slept with them. It was self-defense; that was the only way I could get any sleep.

At the time, I was a medical resident. I had six weeks of maternity leave, and then I went back to working 110 hours a week.

I tried to get my first baby to sleep in his crib. He wouldn't sleep.

## Mommy MD Guides–Recommended Product
### Arm's Reach Mini Arc Convertible

We're all limited by time and money, so products that do double-duty are a mom's dream. The Arm's Reach Mini Arc Convertible actually does *triple* duty, making it even more of a time- and money-saver.

You can use this as a co-sleeper, freestanding bassinet, and play yard. Using it as a co-sleeper lets you reach over and draw your baby close for feeding, comforting, and bonding. It's compact enough to shoe-horn it into your probably already crammed-full bedroom.

Be sure to follow the manufacturer's instructions when using a co-sleeper, or any baby product for that matter. The co-sleeper should fit flush against the parental bed. There must be no more than a $1/2$ inch (13 mm) gap between bedside sleeper and adult bed.

The Mini Arc Convertible comes with a removable fabric liner, mattress, fitted sheet, and travel bag. It folds up so you can take it "to go." You can buy one at **www.ArmsReach.com** for around $100.

A doctor I worked with said, "Do you know that humans are the only mammals that don't sleep with their young? In most countries in the world, even humans sleep with their young. It's only in Western countries where we insist that our babies sleep alone where they can't hear, smell, or see their parents."

After that, I brought my baby in to sleep with me. I took precautions, of course. I wouldn't have been able to sleep if I was worried about my baby. Because I didn't want to sleep too deeply, I drank no alcohol. And I never used any sleep medications.

We eliminated anything in our bed that could cause choking or suffocation. My inclination is to sleep under warm comfy blankets, but I slept in warm pajamas so I could stop using the blankets. I used a very small pillow only the size of my head. I dressed my baby in pajamas and swaddled him tightly in a blanket.

My husband and I didn't sleep with our baby between us. We put a bed rail on my side of the bed, and I slept with the baby between me and the bed rail.

Our babies each slept with us for around four months. I don't think I slept very deeply for that time. But sleeping lightly was preferable to not sleeping at all.

—*Deborah Gilboa, MD, a mom of 14-, 12-, 10-, and 8-year-old sons, a family physician with Squirrel Hill Health Center, in Pittsburgh, PA, and a parenting speaker whose advice is found at AskDoctorG.com*

**A ruffled mind makes a restless pillow.**
—*Charlotte Brontë*

# Chapter 3

## Focusing on Safe Sleeping

Before becoming a mom, you probably didn't think much about safe sleeping. But having a baby truly changes everything. Worrying is part of the mom job description, and whether your little one is awake or sleeping, his safety and well-being are on your mind.

Fortunately, keeping your baby safe at night is far less complicated than keeping him safe when he's awake! You simply set the stage for a safe sleeping environment. Newborns pretty much stay where you put them, so you can feel relatively confident he will stay there. But trust us, that won't be true for long! Enjoy it while it lasts!

### JUSTIFICATION FOR A CELEBRATION

Here's an important safety tip: Create a fire escape plan, including a safe meeting place outside. Practice it often; once a month is great. Have a little celebratory hugging at the meeting place!

> **We sleep safe in our beds because**
> **rough men stand in the night to visit violence**
> **on those who would do us harm.**
>
> —*George Orwell*

## Baby Sleeping Safely

It's so simple: The only thing that should be in your baby's crib with your sleeping little one is a sheet. That's it! Yet, in a study by *American Baby* and Safe Kids Worldwide, nearly three out of four moms admitted to placing at least one item inside the crib with their babies.

- Blanket: 59 percent
- Bumpers: 35 percent
- Stuffed animals: 23 percent
- Pillows: 8 percent

According to the American Academy of Pediatrics (AAP), *all* of the above are suffocation hazards for babies younger than one year old. Having these items in the crib can increase a baby's risk of SIDS up to five times. The risk is so great that the city of Chicago and the state of Maryland have banned the sale of crib bumpers entirely.

Here's a great case for minimalism. Use the baby blankets, stuffies, and pillows as room decorations for now.

### Install Smoke Detectors

You'll sleep more soundly knowing you and your family are safe, and one of the simplest ways to protect your loved ones is to install a smoke alarm on each floor, using lithium batteries that will last for 10 years. Nearly 60 percent of fatal home fires happen in homes without smoke detectors. Taking the simple step of installing the alarms lowers your family's risk of dying in a fire by half, according to the Nemours Foundation.

While you're at it, also install carbon monoxide detectors, which will protect you and your family from carbon monoxide poisoning that occurs when gas is leaked into your home through improperly working heaters, stoves, water heaters, and dryers, along with charcoal grills, running cars, and fireplaces.

**ZZZZz**

## BABY SLEEP PRO TIP: Nap Safely

According to Parents.com, 53 percent of moms sleep on a couch with their infants. This is very risky business.

Your baby should never sleep on a couch or an upholstered chair. This is for several reasons. First, these surfaces are too soft, and a baby sleeping on them is at risk for suffocation. Second, you never know when your baby will roll over for the first time. Murphy's Law dictates that, given the chance, the first time will quite likely be when he's lying on a sofa, rolling over and—right off—onto the floor.

Always put your baby to sleep in a bassinet, crib, cradle, or a bedside co-sleeper, an infant bed that attaches to an adult bed.

**—Rebecca Kempton, MD**

As bad as it sounds, I used a mesh bumper in my baby's crib. This was before they were not recommended. Now I would be sure not to have *any* bumpers in my baby's crib.

> —*Michelle Davis-Dash, MD, a mom of a five-year-old son and a pediatrician, in Baltimore, MD*

When my babies were newborns, they slept in a bassinet in my room. It was only the baby in there—no toys or blankets. Once my babies could roll over, around four months, I introduced a small blanket, but not before.

> —*Eva Mayer, MD, a mom of a 12-year-old daughter and an 11-year-old son, an associate professor of pediatrics at Temple University, and a pediatrician with St. Luke's Hospital Coopersburg Pediatrics, in Pennsylvania*

We didn't have any stuffed toys in the crib with our baby. I didn't want her to roll over onto a toy and not be able to get her face away from it.

Our baby did play with stuffed animals as she got older. Once she was able to push up on her arms and lift her head, I allowed them in her crib with her. When you see that your child can reasonably push up during tummy time and is beginning to crawl, then I think it's okay to have stuffed animals in the crib.

*—Lisa M. Campanella-Coppo, MD, a mom of a six-year-old daughter and an emergency department physician at Summit Medical Group, in Livingston, NJ*

## RALLIE'S TIP

*When my babies were newborns, they slept in cribs with a mattress and nothing else. I had two babies in cribs at once, and the floor of their room was usually a total mess, but I always tried to keep their cribs clear.*

*I dressed my baby boys in temperature-appropriate pajamas so I wouldn't have to worry about them getting tangled up in blankets, which*

### Mommy MD Guides–Recommended Product
#### SwaddleMe Wriggle Blanket

We always used sleep sacks, which are essentially wearable blankets. That way our baby would feel secure and warm in her crib without using loose blankets, which could be dangerous.

—Sonali Ruder, DO, a mom of a three-year-old daughter, an emergency medicine physician, and the author of *Natural Baby Food*, in Fort Lauderdale, FL

The safest way to put your baby to sleep is in a crib that is free of loose blankets. Once your baby "graduates" from a swaddler (See "Summer Infant SwaddleMe" on page 40), consider a sleep sack. You can keep your baby warm and cozy with a Summer Infant SwaddleMeWrap Sack or SwaddleMeWriggle Blanket.

The Wrap Sack gives you a choice of keeping your baby's arms and hands wrapped or free. The Wiggle Blanket is a sleep sack with capped sleeves for warmth. Your baby's arms are still free to move and explore.

Wrap Sacks and Wriggle Blankets don't interfere with your baby's airway, and he won't be able to kick them off. They cost around $19.99. You can buy them at buybuyBaby and other stores nationwide. Visit **SUMMERINFANT.COM** for more information.

*was just one of the hundreds of dangers I obsessed about as a new mother. I had a big, colorful mural on the wall and musical mobiles hanging from the ceiling out of reach so they'd have something to look at.*

*I was never really tempted to keep toys or stuffed animals in my babies' cribs, because I wasn't all that successful at teaching them to stay in their cribs while they were the least bit awake. They were usually nearly asleep when I put them down for a nap or for bedtime. Because I'm an early riser, I usually just went and scooped them up as soon as they started crying or calling for me. So much for self-soothing!*

*The empty crib policy probably made extra work for me and cost me a little sleep, but it was worth it to me knowing that my babies were as safe as they could be. Although I failed to teach my sons to be good self-soothers while they were infants, I'm happy to report that they have all grown up to be strong, independent young men, and they're all able to fall asleep on their own now.*

## Dressing the Baby for Sleep

Few things in life are more delicious than a sleepy, warm, soft, cozy baby dressed in warm, soft, cozy pajamas.

When buying pjs, check the label to see if the fabric is flame-retardant. This means it's been treated with chemicals, which actually you might want to avoid altogether. Used pjs might have been washed so many times that the chemicals are long gone— literally thrown out with the wash water.

If the pajamas haven't been chemically treated, dress your baby in snug-fitting sleepwear. This helps it to be fire-retardant because it minimizes the space between your baby and the clothing.

Consider sleepwear with snaps at the crotch. This will make your life easier when you have to do nighttime diaper changes. Not having to strip the baby naked in the middle of the night is certainly a good thing!

≪∽◦

I dressed my baby for bed in warm pajamas with feet. This way, there was no need for blankets.

—*Michelle Davis-Dash, MD*

## Refer to Your Self-Care Checklist

The constant demands of parenthood can leave you feeling wiped out in a big way, both physically and emotionally. It's common to hear new mothers (well, honestly, any mothers) say they forgot to eat or have no time for a shower because they're so busy taking care of the baby. But self-care is as important as the care you give your baby. You'll be a happier, healthier parent when you take the time to take care of yourself, and you'll teach your child to value self-care as she grows older.

Make a checklist of self-care basics and ask yourself if you're hitting every one of them daily or regularly. If not, try working them into your schedule. Here's what to include on your checklist. Add in others you feel are important.

- Eat nutritious meals three times a day.

- Take time for a shower or to wash your face and moisturize.

- Get some exercise almost every day of the week.

- Keep up your doctors' appointments.

- Get outside for fresh air and sunshine.

- Carve out special, romantic, private time for your husband or partner.

- Socialize with friends and family.

- Vent to a friend or family member about your frustrations.

- Get quiet time to read, write in a journal, or simply sit and reflect on your life.

- Take time for your spiritual health by meditating, going to church, or joining a spiritual group.

- Do something special for yourself, such as getting a haircut, massage, manicure, pedicure, or facial.

- Take a class to learn a new hobby or to do something you already enjoy, such as cooking or painting.

- Get to bed early.

I always dressed my babies, especially my newborns, in as many layers as I wore, plus one thin additional layer. This simple rule ensures that the baby isn't overdressed or underdressed. Neither is good for a baby. For their first three months, I dressed them in a diaper, undershirt, and pajamas, swaddled in a light blanket.

> —Hana R. Solomon, MD, *a mom of four grown biological children, two grown "spiritually adopted" children, a grandmom of eight, a pediatrician, the president of BeWell Health, LLC, the inventor of Dr. Hana's Nasopure nose wash for children, and the author of* Clearing the Air One Nose at a Time: Caring for Your Personal Filter, *the owner's manual for the nose, in Columbia, MO*

I wanted to avoid blankets in the crib. To make sure my babies were warm enough, I dressed them in one layer more than I was wearing, such as a onesie and footed pajamas.

> —Kristy Magee, MD, *a mom of 15-, 12-, and 8-year-old sons and a family physician at North Seminole Family Practice and Sports Medicine, in Sanford, FL*

My kids are all partial to wearing soft, comfortable clothing. I am too! My kids tend to wear pajamas and sleepers that are soft and cotton. I try to make sure all of their sleepwear is cotton because polyester can get so hot and uncomfortable during the night.

> —Sigrid Payne DaVeiga, MD, *a mom of 10-year-old and 1-month-old sons and a 5-year-old daughter and a pediatric allergist with the Children's Hospital of Philadelphia, in Pennsylvania*

For the first 12 to 15 months of both my children's lives, I used sleep sacks on top of their pajamas to keep them cozy while they slept. We did not keep any blankets in their cribs with them.

> —Manpreet K. Gill, MD, *a mom of a five-year-old daughter and a three-year-old son and a family practice physician with North Seminole Family Practice, in Sanford, FL*

My grandkids have special sleep sacks that they wear to bed. These are great because they're snuggly.

Also because their feet are in the sack, they can't stand and get enough traction to fling themselves out of the crib—as my second child did.

*—Kathryn Boling, MD, a mom of two grown daughters, a grandmom of two, and a family medicine physician with Mercy Medical Center, in Baltimore, MD*

## Mommy MD Guides-Recommended Product
### Snuza Baby Movement Monitor

We used a Snuza for the baby. This device fits on the baby's diaper and detects breathing.

SIDS was our biggest fear in the first 18 months. The causes of SIDS are still poorly understood, and we wanted to do everything we could to minimize our baby's risk. Knowing that my baby was wearing a Snuza put my mind at ease, so I could get some sleep too! The Snuza is the only item we used that helped me get a decent night's sleep.

—Edna Ma, MD, a mom of a 4-year-old son and an 18-month-old daughter, an anesthesiologist, and the founder of BareEASE pre-waxing numbing kit, in Los Angeles, CA

Snuza baby movement monitors measure the baby's breathing through her abdominal movement. In the most recent model, PICO, it also monitors, body temperature and her position, and streams the information to your smartphone or tablet. The manufacturer offers three baby movement monitors: Snuza Go! for $99.99, Snuza Hero for $119.99, and its latest and smallest monitor, Snuza Pico for $139.99.

You can buy the monitors at Babies R Us, Buy Buy Baby, Target, and other retailers nationwide. For more information about Snuza, visit **SNUZA.COM**.

I dressed our babies in light, long-sleeved cotton onesies. But I worried that they might get cold in the night, so I put them in zipper sleep sacks. They're like mini sleeping bags.

—*Marcela Dominguez, MD, a mom of a 13-year-old daughter and an 11-year-old son who has a private family medicine and wellness practice in Southern California, whose concierge medicine services are provided by Signature MD*

෴

For my babies' first four to six weeks, I put infant hats on them at night to sleep. You want to use a very soft hat that's well fitted—the type you might have gotten from the hospital.

Babies' heads are bigger compared to their bodies. If your baby's head is uncovered, he can lose a lot of body heat through his head and get hypothermia. Babies need to use all of the energy from breast milk or formula to grow and develop. You don't want your baby to have to "waste" that energy staying warm.

—*Aline T. Tanios Keyrouz, MD, a mom of 13- and 7-year-old and 9-month-old daughters and an 11-year-son and an assistant professor of pediatrics at St. Louis University, in Missouri*

## Putting the Baby to Sleep on His Back

Sudden Infant Death Syndrome (SIDS) is the leading cause of death in infants between one month and one year of age. A risk for SIDS is babies sleeping on their stomachs. Yet more than a quarter of moms say they've put their babies to sleep on their stomachs.

There's no middle ground here either. Side sleeping isn't recommended because it's too great a risk for the baby to roll over onto her stomach.

Way back in 1992, the American Academy of Pediatrics (AAP) first recommended that all babies be placed on their backs to sleep. In the quarter century since, deaths from SIDS have declined dramatically.

*Always* put your baby "back to sleep."

We always were careful to put our babies to sleep on their backs to reduce their risk of SIDS.

—*Shilpa Amin-Shah, MD, a mom of a 6-year-old son and 5-year-old and 18-month-old daughters and an emergency medicine physician at Emergency Medical Associates, in St. Johns, FL*

❧

When my baby was a newborn, my mom came to visit. She insisted on putting him on his tummy to sleep because of his gastric reflux. It took me a while to get him out of that habit. I just consistently laid him down to sleep on his back, and he adjusted to that again.

—*Michelle Davis-Dash, MD*

❧

I always put my babies to sleep on their backs. But I noticed that sometimes if they were flat on their backs, they'd get fussy. They might have had a little reflux. Those nights, I took a small towel, rolled it up, and tucked it underneath the crib mattress. This raised up one side of the mattress just enough so that the baby's head was slightly higher—not enough for her to roll over onto her stomach.

—*Lauren Hyman, MD, a mom of a 13-year-old daughter and an 11-year-old son and an ob-gyn at West Hills Hospital and Medical Center, in California*

❧

When my babies were newborns, I always put them to sleep on their backs. I worried that they might vomit and aspirate it into their lungs.

To prevent that from happening, I elevated the head of the mattress a bit. I placed a rolled-up towel under the mattress. This way, gravity helped to keep them from aspirating if they vomited. This is also helpful for babies with congestion or reflux.

—*Eva Mayer, MD, a mom of a 12-year-old daughter and an 11-year-old son, an associate professor of pediatrics at Temple University, and a pediatrician with St. Luke's Hospital Coopersburg Pediatrics, in Pennsylvania*

## Monitoring the Baby's Sleep

Baby monitors run the gamut—from light-sleeping husbands nudging moms awake to products like iBabyGuard that detects and actively displays your baby's breath count on your Apple and Android devices. (Big mother is watching you…)

The type of monitor that appeals to you probably says a lot about your mothering style. More casual, less nervous moms might prefer a simple no-frills sound monitor. (Can you hear me now?) Moms who like more contact and direct observation of their wee ones probably would rather have a sound *and* video monitor.

Newer "next-gen" monitors can sense all sorts of things, such as your baby's movements, breathing, activity level, and body position. Some of these products provide sleep alerts, and they can even generate nightly reports on your baby's sleep. (But really what new mom has the energy to read them?)

*All* monitors can give moms some peace of mind—and some space of mind when they need to do something—anything!—while the baby is napping.

⤞⤝

We used a video monitor in our baby's room. The Motorola monitor was inexpensive, had a great picture quality, and played lullabies.
—*Shilpa Amin-Shah, MD*

⤞⤝

We always had a sound monitor in our babies' rooms, but not a video monitor. As I am with any electronic device, I would've been glued to a video monitor. It's like feeling compelled to check your smartphone.

Also, when you have just a sound monitor, I think a mommy learns to recognize what her baby's different cries mean, and this allows you to respond accordingly.
—*Antoinette Cheney, DO, a mom of a 12-year-old son and an 11-year-old daughter, a family physician with Rocky Vista University College of Osteopathic Medicine, in Parker, CO*

I used a sound monitor in my baby's room. I felt that hearing my baby was enough. I also think that if the child is quietly resting during naptime and you don't hear anything, then you should both take the much-needed respite.

The video monitors don't allow for that. I have seen people become obsessed with them, watching their child's every move. I have a close relative who would watch her daughter play for the entire hour of naptime and get so frustrated that she would go and take her out of her crib.

## Mommy MD Guides–Recommended Product
### Graco Secure Coverage Digital Monitor with Two Parent Units

I used a Graco sound monitor when my kids were babies. I remember one day, I was cooking in the kitchen. Over the monitor, I heard my daughter, who was three at the time, tell my son, who was one at the time, "Here! You put your leg over the side of the crib here to climb out!" After that, there were no more cribs for them!
> —Eva Mayer, MD, a mom of a 12-year-old daughter and an 11-year-old son, an associate professor of pediatrics at Temple University, and a pediatrician with St. Luke's Hospital Coopersburg Pediatrics, in Pennsylvania

The Secure Coverage Digital Monitor uses digital technology that, according to the manufacturer, is secure and private, while offering a range of 2,000 feet and 900 MHz frequency so it doesn't get interference from other electronics. In addition to helping you hear the smallest noises from your baby, the monitor will vibrate when he calls for you. You can clip it to your belt to carry with you.

The monitor with two parent units costs $64.99 and can be bought directly from Graco's website, **GracoBaby.com**, or from mass-market retailers.

I think it's best to have your child get used to having a period of daily quiet time even if he doesn't actually sleep. This gives you a period of time when you can take a break.

—*Lisa M. Campanella-Coppo, MD*

⟡

My mom came to visit after my first child was born. Mom is a card-carrying member of the "Greatest Generation," who endured the Great Depression and WWII, raised seven of us rugrats, including one who was severely disabled, all while being a successful entrepreneur and author. (Can you understand my "wonder woman" complex?!) Mom took one look at the baby monitor and asked, "What's that?"

I said, "It's a monitor. So you can hear the baby cry."

My mom's completely serious response was, "Why would you want to?"

—*Susan Wilder, MD, a mom of a 22-year-old daughter and 17-year-old twins, a primary care physician, and the founder and CEO of LifeScape Premier, LLC, in Scottsdale, AZ*

⟡

I'm old school. We didn't use a baby monitor. I just slept lightly and used my ears. When my kids were babies, there were no video monitors, and the audio ones weren't that reliable. Sometimes they would transmit random radio sounds!

—*Susan Besser, MD, a mom of six grown children, a grandmom of five, and a family physician at River Family Physicians, in Easton, MD*

⟡

We didn't have a monitor for our babies. We didn't need one. We lived in a small cottage with hardwood floors, and our bedroom was located between our kids' bedrooms, so we could hear them plenty well.

—*Marcela Dominguez, MD*

# Chapter 4

## Making the Conditions Right for Sleep

According to the National Sleep Foundation, adults spend quite a lot of time and energy making the conditions right for sleep.

- 93 percent of Americans say having a good mattress is key to a good night's sleep.
- 91 percent say they change their sheets at least every other week.
- 78 percent say they like their sheets to have a fresh scent.
- 73 percent say a dark bedroom is important for a good night's sleep.
- 74 percent say a quiet room is important.

We bet that 100 percent of parents say that having your baby sleep is critical to a good night's sleep. So setting the stage for your baby's sleep is very important.

But bear in mind, you can make all of the conditions just right, but you can't make your baby sleep!

### JUSTIFICATION FOR A CELEBRATION

Practice makes perfect for most things, including swaddling. When you perfect your swaddling technique so well that your little Houdini can't escape, that's plenty of reason to celebrate!

> ### Hot Water Bottles
> It's quaint and old-fashioned, but placing a hot water bottle at your feet or wearing socks will improve circulation and elevate your body temperature.

## Swaddling the Baby for Sleep

One of the hardest parts of being a mom is making the best, safest choices for your children. This is often complicated by changing, conflicting medical advice and media reports.

Case in point is the May 2016 *Pediatrics* study that questioned the safety of swaddling and implicated swaddling in increased risk of Sudden Infant Death Syndrome (SIDS).

In our Tweet-length–attention-span world, the nuances of studies like these are quickly lost. To make matters worse, over-simplified, headline-grabbing sound bites don't come anywhere close to telling the full story. Here are important points to understand.

• This study was a *review* of a handful of previously published studies. It didn't include new research designed to study swaddling in depth.

• The studies didn't clearly define "swaddling." It's not possible to know if the babies who died of SIDS were swaddled safely and correctly and using products made specifically for swaddling—or if these babies had been "swaddled" incorrectly.

• One of the findings of the study is that babies are at risk for SIDS when they sleep on their stomachs. This was already a clearly established risk—and it's a risk whether a baby is swaddled or not.

So often in parenting, as in life, the best advice is to "stay the course." Mothers have instinctively swaddled their babies, generation after generation. Babies are born from completely warm, safe, comforting wombs into a cold, new world. Swaddling helps babies experience the comfort and sense of security that they had in the womb.

⁓

I always swaddled my babies like little burritos. It helped them to sleep better.

—*Antoinette Cheney, DO, a mom of a 12-year-old son and an 11-year-old daughter, and a family physician with Rocky Vista University College of Osteopathic Medicine, in Parker, CO*

We swaddled our daughter when she was a baby. But she liked to fling her arms out to her sides. She could get out of our swaddling like a mini Houdini! I think that she enjoyed having her space.

—*Katja Rowell, MD, a mom of a 10-year-old daughter, a family practice physician, and the author of* Helping Your Child with Extreme Picky Eating *and* Love Me, Feed Me *at thefeedingdoctor.com, in St Paul, MN*

My husband and I found that swaddling my daughter tightly was the best option. Swaddling was absolutely key to getting good sleep.

We started swaddling almost from day one. We had cotton baby

## Mommy MD Guides–Recommended Product
### Summer Infant SwaddleMe

We swaddled our newborn with the Summer Infant SwaddleMe. I loved the material.

SwaddleMe blankets replace loose blankets in the crib. They also help keep babies sleeping safely on their backs. Because swaddling re-creates the snugness of the womb, babies startle themselves awake less, and they stay asleep longer.

—Shilpa Amin-Shah, MD, a mom of a 6-year-old son and 5-year-old and 18-month-old daughters and an emergency medicine physician at Emergency Medical Associates, in St. Johns, FL

Swaddling helps your baby feel cozy and safe like she did in the womb and allows you to put your baby to bed safely with a blanket. Summer Infant SwaddleMe blankets come in different sizes to keep your baby wrapped up snug, and you can choose from a variety of colors and patterns.

A single SwaddleMe original swaddle blanket costs $14.99 and can be purchased at retailers and baby stores nationwide, or on Summer Infant's website at **SummerInfant.com**.

blankets that we would fold in half in a triangle, and then we would put her on it with the point at her feet and her neck lined up with the straight edge. The point was folded up and then the sides were wrapped around her. The key was that her arms had to be tucked in and everything had to be snug. This also served a second purpose in that it kept her from scratching her face with her nails.

As our daughter got a bit older, we'd leave her arms out.

—*Lisa M. Campanella-Coppo, MD, a mom of a six-year-old daughter and an emergency department physician at Summit Medical Group, in Livingston, NJ*

I love soft baby blankets; I've found my favorites at Target and Home Goods. Also, Aden + Anais makes some very soft swaddling blankets that I love as well. (See Mommy MD Guides–Recommended Product on page 124.)

Recently after my newborn's birth, I had a conversation with a nursery nurse who explained to me the importance of swaddling. It really struck a chord with me. She described how none of the baby's movements are directed in any way in these early days. It's very comforting for babies to feel swaddled or bundled because they just left such a tight space in the womb.

My son is almost two months old now, and he still appreciates being swaddled. A baby's startle reflexes always look so jarring and unsettling to me. I think swaddling in the first couple of months is very helpful.

—*Sigrid Payne DaVeiga, MD, a mom of 10-year-old and 1-month-old sons and a 5-year-old daughter and a pediatric allergist with the Children's Hospital of Philadelphia, in Pennsylvania*

I swaddled all four of my babies. I used a blanket. You can swaddle a baby with any square or rectangular blanket.

Here's how to swaddle: Lay the blanket on a flat surface such as the floor with one corner up, like a diamond. Fold the top corner down. Place your baby so the fold is at the nape of his neck. Pull one side of the blanket up and over your baby and firmly tuck it under his side. Fold the bottom up. Pull the other side of the blanket up and over your baby and firmly tuck it underneath him.

Swaddling your baby like this re-creates the womb-like feeling. Swaddling was the one thing that helped my kids sleep for their first few months.

—*Deborah Gilboa, MD, a mom of 14-, 12-, 10-, and 8-year-old sons, a family physician with Squirrel Hill Health Center, in Pittsburgh, PA, and a parenting speaker whose advice is found at AskDoctorG.com*

I liked the SwaddleMe swaddler because it has a two-way zipper.

—*Sonali Ruder, DO, a mom of a three-year-old daughter, an emergency medicine physician, and the author of* Natural Baby Food, *in Fort Lauderdale, FL*

## Controlling the Noise

Country music–loving adults might love to hear Kenny Chesney sing about "Noise," but when there's a baby in the house, new moms often become quite obsessed with controlling it. It can be difficult to keep the household noise at that Goldilocks level—not too soft, not too loud, *just* right.

It's pretty much a parenting rite of passage: Just when you finally get your baby off to slumberland, a firetruck goes screaming down the street, a glass bowl slips through your fingers to the floor with a crash, or the house phone rings!

We had two dogs that would bark at everything, so our house was never quiet. I always felt this was an advantage because now my kids can sleep through anything.

—*Jeannette Gonzalez Simon, DO, a mom of seven- and five-year-old daughters and a pediatric gastroenterologist, in Verona, NJ*

With my first baby, we were super quiet. With my second, we didn't even try to be quiet. Now he can fall asleep literally anywhere. He can sleep through anything, even fire alarms. (See "Mommy MD Guides-Recommended Product: Nest Protect Smoke Alarm" on page 41.)

—*Heather Orman-Lubell, MD, a mom of 15- and 11-year-old sons and a pediatrician at St. Chris Care at Yardley Pediatrics, in Pennsylvania*

We never made much effort to be quiet for our babies to sleep. After all, it's not quiet in the womb! Babies constantly hear the noises of their mothers' heart, intestines, and lungs.

Ours is a full house with two adults and four children and often a nanny and her two children. We never were quiet, and as a result, our children can still sleep easily regardless of whether I have people over or whether we are going in and out for work.

—*Rebecca Jeanmonod, MD, a mom of 12- and 8-year-old daughters and 11- and 8-year-old sons and a professor of emergency medicine and the associate residency program director for the emergency medicine residency at St. Luke's University Health Network, in Bethlehem, PA*

**BABY SLEEP PRO TIP:** Use White Noise

Set your baby up for sleep success by adding some white noise, like the sound of a shower or a fan. Re-creating the whooshing sounds from the womb is comforting and sleep-inducing. Even toddlers and adults benefit from white noise. A fan works well, and there are many free white noise apps, such as Relax Melodies.

**—Rebecca Kempton, MD**

Before they are born, babies are "serenaded" with their mothers' steady heartbeat. So after babies are born, they feel best with mom's heartbeat and other sounds nearby.

I hope that all parents, grandparents, aunts, uncles, and cousins speak, sing, and touch mom's pregnant belly (if appropriate) so the entire village can bond with the baby. When the baby is born, the extended family will feel more bonded, and the baby will know their voices. I tried this with my latest grandbaby. I've been spending hours cooing, singing, and making eye contact with him. Just three days short of three weeks of age, my grandbaby consistently responds with smiles when he hears my voice!

—*Hana R. Solomon, MD, a mom of four grown biological children, two grown "spiritually adopted" children, a grandmom of eight, a pediatrician, the president of BeWell Health, LLC, the inventor of Dr. Hana's Nasopure nose wash for children, and the author of* Clearing the Air One Nose at a Time: Caring for Your Personal Filter, *the owner's manual for the nose, in Columbia, MO*

In my baby's nursery, we used a sleep machine that sounded like waves. We also always had the fan on—both for air circulation to help control the temperature as well as to mute any outside noise.

—*Kathryn Boling, MD, a mom of two grown daughters, a grandmom of two, and a family medicine physician with Mercy Medical Center, in Baltimore, MD*

When our daughter was a very young baby, we didn't try to keep quiet at all. She slept right through it all. As she got older, that changed, and we used a white noise machine.

—*Katja Rowell, MD*

⁓

In my baby's room, I used a fan as white noise. It helped to signal bedtime and create a calming environment.

—*Mona Gohara, MD, a mom of nine- and seven-year-old sons, a dermatologist in private practice, in Danbury, CT, and an associate clinical professor in the department of dermatology at Yale University*

⁓

At night, I wanted my kids' rooms to be quiet for sleeping, but at naptime I played classical music for them. Research suggests that music could help with babies' cognitive development.

—*Kristy Magee, MD, a mom of 15-, 12-, and 8-year-old sons and a family physician at North Seminole Family Practice and Sports Medicine, in Sanford, FL*

⁓

When my boys were babies, I played classical music for them on CD. They still enjoy it today. In fact, when I say it's time to settle down, they will find classical music on the iPod and listen to it.

—*Sharon Boyce, MD, a mom of seven- and five-year-old sons and a family physician with Oaklawn Medical Group, in Albion and Bellevue, MI*

## Breathe in the Soothing Scents of Essential Oils

**MomMy TIME** Create an environment in your bedroom ideal for sleep through aromatherapy, the practice of using essential oils. Lavender and chamomile oils help bring on relaxation, while eucalyptus can open congested nasal passages for more restful sleep. Essential oils can be combined with a base oil and rubbed onto the skin, added to a bowl of steaming water to be inhaled, placed into a warm bath, or used with a diffuser.

> "If we wish to have a beautiful, peaceful,
> and safe home, we need healthy expanding roots
> that go deep into the ground. These roots are
> our routine, our stability, our structure."
>
> —*Natasa Pantovic Nuit,* Conscious Parenting

When my kids were babies, we had a Fisher-Price aquarium that hung on the inside of the crib. It really helped. Even at around six months old, they could tap it at night and it would play music. It was a great transitional object. Sometimes in the middle of the night, I would hear the aquarium start to play, and I knew my baby had woken up and tapped it.

> —*Eva Mayer, MD, a mom of a 12-year-old daughter and an 11-year-old son, an associate professor of pediatrics at Temple University, and a pediatrician with St. Luke's Hospital Coopersburg Pediatrics, in Pennsylvania*

When my daughter was a baby, we used a Sleep Sheep, which is a white noise machine in a cute stuffed animal. It has a few different settings, and we would attach it to the outside of my daughter's crib. It has an automatic shut-off so it turns off after a set amount of time.

I found that my daughter liked the white noise settings as well as the sound of a heartbeat, which is supposed to make babies feel like they're back in the womb. It seemed to help her sleep better.

> —*Sonali Ruder, DO*

I didn't play any music or white noise while my baby slept. I didn't want him to get accustomed to it and need it to fall to sleep. This worked well for my family.

> —*Michelle Davis-Dash, MD, a mom of a five-year-old son and a pediatrician, in Baltimore, MD*

When our babies were around six weeks old, they moved out of the bassinet in our room to their own room with a crib. We're "basic" parents. We had simple, comfortable rooms for them. We didn't go to any extremes with white noise, but we did have dimming light.

—*Marcela Dominguez, MD, a mom of a 13-year-old daughter and an 11-year-old son who has a private family medicine and wellness practice in Southern California, whose concierge medicine services are provided by Signature MD*

## Mommy MD Guides-Recommended Product
### Cloud B Giraffe

When my twins were babies, we used a white noise machine—Cloud B Gentle Giraffe Plush Sound Machine with Four Soothing Sounds. Later we switched to a HEPA air filter that also substitutes for white noise. I love the white noise. It's especially important because my twins are light sleepers, and our house can be noisy!
—Sonal R. Patel, MD, a mom of four-year-old twin daughters and a physician who specializes in pediatric/adult allergy and immunology with Adventist Health Physicians Network, in Los Angeles, CA

Cloud B offers sleep toys that can soothe your baby through sight, sound, scent, or touch. Sound toys include plush toys such as a sheep, owl, frog, giraffe, turtle, fox, and a host of other animals that contain a hidden sound box that your child can activate to play melodies. If your baby prefers soothing warmth and scent instead of sound, the Cloud B Cozies Turtle or Sheep includes a lavender wheat heat pack.

The toys cost from $14.99 to $54.95, depending on which one you choose. You can buy them at **CloudB.com/US/Shop**.

I tried not to "fake" my babies' sleeping environments any more than I had to. Because of this, my fourth son could pretty much sleep anywhere.

This kid liked chaos so much he practically *needed* it to sleep. I have a great picture of him at overnight camp: In the dining room with 350 kids, my son was stretched out fast asleep on a picnic bench.

We used to joke that when my son was breastfeeding, if there wasn't a lot of noise and chaos, he'd stop nursing and look around as if he was thinking, *What's up? I ordered dinner* and *a show!*

—*Deborah Gilboa, MD*

Both of our children used a Cloud B Giraffe projector with lights and music in their cribs in their first year. This helped to signal to them that it was time to sleep. It helped to add a soothing, calming effect to their sleep environment. (See "Cloud B Giraffe" on page 47.)

—*Manpreet K. Gill, MD, a mom of a five-year-old daughter and a three-year-old son and a family practice physician with North Seminole Family Practice, in Sanford, FL*

## Tweaking the Temperature

"The woods are lovely, dark, and deep, but I have miles to go before I sleep." Turns out if those woods are a little chilly, Robert Frost might have just dropped to the ground and slept anyway. A mild drop in body temperature induces your body to sleep.

At nighttime, set the temperature in your home between 60 and 67 degrees Fahrenheit, the ideal sleeping temperature for adults. A higher—or lower—temperature can make you restless and even wreck the quality of your rapid eye movement (REM) sleep.

Because the core body temperature needs to drop in order to fall asleep, I maintained my baby's room temperature between 68 and 70 degrees, monitored with our thermostat.

—*Rebecca Kempton, MD, a mom of eight- and six-year-old sons and a three-year-old-daughter and an infant and toddler sleep specialist, in Chicago, IL*

I kept the temperature in my baby's room at 68 degrees Fahrenheit. I kept a small rotating fan on for both the background noise and also to circulate air.

Now my daughter is 18 months old, and she still sleeps with a fan on. We also use a cool mist humidifier during naps and sleep.

*—Shilpa Amin-Shah, MD, a mom of 6-year-old son and 5-year and 18-month old daughters and an emergency medicine physician at Emergency Medical Associates, in St. Johns, FL*

We kept the temperature the same throughout the house in living areas and in our bedroom as well as in our baby's bedroom. If we were comfortable, we assumed the baby was comfortable. But he was swaddled for the first four months.

If he ever woke up sweating, we would cool it down in the house.

*—Nilong Parikh Vyas, MD, MPH, a mom of seven- and five-year-old sons and the founder and owner of Sleepless in NOLA sleep consulting, in New Orleans, LA*

We didn't adjust the temperature in our home or bedrooms when our babies were born. We wanted them to adjust to us, rather than vice versa.

*—Deborah Gilboa, MD*

**BABY SLEEP PRO TIP:** Maintain Cool Room Temperature

Don't let your baby overheat during sleep. Core body temperature must dip in order to fall asleep, so don't overdress your baby for bedtime.

Of course, you don't want her to be too cold either. Aim for a room temperature of about 68 to 72 degrees Fahrenheit, and dress your baby in a single layer of clothing topped by a sleep sack.

A fan can be helpful to circulate air. Place it out of reach and face it away from the crib. Use of fans has been shown to reduce SIDS risk by as much as 72 percent.

**—Rebecca Kempton, MD**

## Lighting Up the Dark

You might want to light up your baby's life, but don't do this at night! Our bodies need the cue of darkness to sleep properly. In fact your body is programmed to sleep when it's dark.

❧

Darkness is what activates melatonin, our internal sleep hormone, and so my baby's room was cave like. Black garbage bags taped over windows can work wonders!

—*Rebecca Kempton, MD, a mom of eight- and six-year-old sons and a three-year-old daughter and an infant and toddler sleep specialist, in Chicago, IL*

❧

We kept the baby's room dark, but we had a nightlight in the hall for parent safety when we were walking in and out. As our daughter got older, we needed to put a nightlight in her room so she wouldn't bump into things or fall if she got out of bed during the night.

—*Lisa M. Campanella-Coppo, MD*

### Mommy MD Guides-Recommended Product
#### Light Projectors

For my grandkids, we have a combination sleep machine that also projects images onto the ceiling: stars, jungle cartoon animals, and fish. It's very soothing and hypnotizing.

Wherever my grandkids go, they need that machine to sleep. It helps them relax, and when the machine is playing, it is a trigger to get sleepy. Works like a charm. Wish they'd had that when my kids were little.

—Kathryn Boling, MD

Soothe your baby to sleep with a gizmo that projects light on the ceiling and plays lullabies, white noise, or nature sounds. You'll find several different types of projectors in stores and online. They cost around $25 and can be found at massmarket retailers.

## Invest in Sleep Gear

Using blackout curtains, eye shades, ear plugs, "white noise machines, fans, and other devices can dissipate any light and noises that can disturb your sleep.

Both of my kids have alarm clocks in their rooms. But even the light emitted from a digital clock can interfere with sleep.

I always set a small object, such as a book, in front of the display to block the light. My kids can simply move it to the side to check the time.

—*Lauren Hyman, MD, a mom of a 13-year-old daughter and an 11-year-old son and an ob-gyn at West Hills Hospital and Medical Center, in California*

As it got closer to bedtime, I exposed my babies to less and less light. Bright light tells your body it's time to wake up; low light tells your body it's time to sleep. Screen time can be particularly disruptive to sleep. Make sure not to expose your child to iPads, smartphones, or televisions for at least an hour before bedtime.

—*Eva Ritvo, MD, a mom of two grown daughters, a psychiatrist, and a coauthor of* The Beauty Prescription, *in Miami Beach, FL*

When my babies were young, I mostly had a nightlight either in the bedroom or in the hall. I didn't want my children to be trained to sleep only in pure darkness, because that is frequently difficult to achieve. Also because my kids doubled up in bedrooms, and because of age differences, one might go to sleep while the other was still awake and reading or doing homework. That made having a dark room impossible.

—*Susan Besser, MD, a mom of six grown children, a grandmom of five, and a family physician at River Family Physicians, in Easton, MD*

*ZZZzz*

**BABY SLEEP PRO TIP:** Darken the Room

Make the room pitch black. Turn off closet lights, nightlights, and block that light seeping in from the sides of the blinds as much as possible. Even black garbage bags work in a pinch. The darkness is what helps the release of our internal sleep hormone, melatonin, so the darker the better.

**—Rebecca Kempton, MD**

To make my baby's room dark, we put up blackout shades. The room was pitch black during the day as well as at night, with the exception of a nightlight. You want your baby to be able to see where he is when he goes to sleep as well as when he wakes up, without it being too dark.

—*Nilong Parikh Vyas, MD, MPH*

> **No day is so bad it can't be fixed with a nap.**
> —*Carrie Snow, stand-up comedian*

# Chapter 5

## Establishing a Routine

It's common knowledge that children thrive on routine. Less well known is that many moms do too. As the pace of life accelerates, sometimes a routine is the crazy glue keeping it all from coming apart at the seams.

Everyone from your mother-in-law, to your pediatrician, to the saleslady at Sleepy's will advise you to get your baby on a nighttime routine. While you're at it, get yourself on one too. If you have your own bedtime ritual to distance yourself from the stressful events of the day, it can get your body and mind ready for sleep.

While it's best for your baby's routine to be simple—bath, books, bed—we encourage you to make yours as fun and elaborate as you'd like. Extra points for alliteration! How about wine, whine (to husband), and more wine.

### JUSTIFICATION FOR A CELEBRATION
One glorious day, your routine runs like Amtrak!

> *There is a time for many words,*
> *and there is also a time for sleep.*
>
> *—Homer, The Odyssey*

## Consider the Tried and True

When your baby is about six weeks old, his sleep patterns begin to emerge. (Is that a cheer we hear?) If you haven't already established a predictable, consistent bedtime routine, this is the perfect time to really start.

It's hard to go wrong with the tried and true—and might we add great alliteration!—of bath, books, bed!

**BABY SLEEP PRO TIP:** Establish Bedtime Routines

Bedtime routines are a key aspect of establishing healthy sleep habits. They can be implemented from the very beginning when your baby comes home from the hospital. Here are some tips to creating a cozy, effective bedtime routine:

• **Start early.** By the time your baby is eight weeks old, establish a consistent bedtime routine that you can repeat before each sleep period—both bedtime and naps.

• **Be predictable and consistent.** Doing the same routine, in the same order, for every sleep period will help your baby to learn to associate the bedtime routine with sleep.

• **Allow anyone to do it.** Help your baby to become a flexible sleeper by enlisting others to help with the routine. Even if you are nursing, your husband or partner can take over after a feeding for the remainder of the routine.

• **Feed then read.** Many babies develop a very strong nurse/bottle to sleep association that can cause night wakings. To help break this association, shift the feeding before the routine (even in a different space) followed by the remainder of the routine—such as books, massage, and singing lullabies—in the bedroom.

• **Be creative.** Allow 15 to 20 minutes for the routine, and do it in the same order, but anything goes! Here are some ideas: Give a gentle massage with lotion, read books, sing some lullabies, make up poems or short stories, and hold your baby and do a slow dance to music.

—*Rebecca Kempton, MD*

Our daughter never wanted to go to sleep! Our pediatrician suggested
that we get into a nightly routine: bath time, lotion, read a few books,
and then bedtime. It took some time, but after a while it worked. Once
we finished the last page of the book, our daughter would roll over and
close her eyes. She knew it was bedtime!

— *Sonali Ruder, DO, a mom of a three-year-old daughter, an
emergency medicine physician, and the author of* Natural Baby
Food, *in Fort Lauderdale, FL*

Our routine has always been: bath, massage, books, bed.

We start early each day, and we have an established routine
we try to maintain. Bath time starts at 5:45 pm, books at 6 pm, and in
bed by 6:15 pm.

— *Shilpa Amin-Shah, MD, a mom of a 6-year-old son and
5-year-old and 18-month-old daughters and an emergency medicine
physician at Emergency Medical Associates, in St. Johns, FL*

Every night, my kids have a bath. I am a fan of the California Baby
products, especially the Calming Shampoo and Body Wash. After
bath, we apply a moisturizer, such as Mustela, which has such a nice
fragrance, or we use good old Vaseline on particularly dry areas.

Then my kids get into some cozy pajamas and slippers, and we
settle down on the couch to read or watch a favorite TV show together.
My daughter, now five years old, is a big fan of *Cupcake Wars*, so we
watch a piece of an old episode every night before she starts to doze
off and then moves to her bed.

— *Sigrid Payne DaVeiga, MD, a mom of 10-year-old and
1-month-old sons and a 5-year-old daughter and a pediatric allergist
with the Children's Hospital of Philadelphia, in Pennsylvania*

I tried to listen to my baby's internal clock—feed him when he's hungry, let him sleep when he's tired—work his routines and patterns into a routine that works for everyone else in the family, and establish a bedtime that makes sense for everyone. I think there should be a reasonable bedtime. You don't need to collapse or be terribly tired in order to go to bed around your bedtime.

—*Ayala Laufer-Cahana, MD, a mom of 20- and 18-year-old sons and a 17-year-old daughter, a pediatrician, artist, entrepreneur, and founder of Herbal Water Inc. and DrAyala .com, in greater Philadelphia, PA*

Nighttime routines are extremely important. Our brains love routine!

When you start a bedtime routine for your baby, the best thing to do is to set a pattern that you can keep consistent. The goal is to make a calming routine—not re-energize them!

I set regular sleeping and waking times. I gave my babies a warm bath after they had the chance to digest their dinner.

—*Eva Ritvo, MD, a mom of two grown daughters, a psychiatrist, and a coauthor of* The Beauty Prescription, *in Miami Beach, FL*

Our kiddo was on the bigger side, and she slept about six hours a night from the time she was eight weeks old. She did that the first night we tried a bedtime ritual, so we stuck with it.

We used a space heater to pre-warm the bathroom. We gave her a warm bath (no soap, just warm water), then we would use a safe massage oil and give her a body massage for about 10 to 15 minutes. (I had taken an infant massage class.) We put her in cozy jammies and then cuddled her with a final bottle, and then we put her in her crib to sleep. She went in her crib awake most of the time. Many nights she cried softly for a minute or two, but then she went to sleep.

I worried initially about the crying, but she slept well, self-soothed for a time (that changed when she was about 15 months old), and always woke with a huge smile! I know that some of her success with sleep was our routine, but probably most was her temperament and sleep style. I think it helps parents to know that what works for one baby might not work for another. Some babies just have an easier time with sleep than others.

—*Katja Rowell, MD, a mom of a 10-year-old daughter, a family practice physician, and the author of* Helping Your Child with Extreme Picky Eating and Love Me, Feed Me *at TheFeedingDoctor.com, in St. Paul, MN*

Here's a parenting secret: You have to *establish* a bedtime routine when your kids are babies in order for it to actually *work* when they are toddlers.

Because I have four children, when they were little, I did their bedtime routine in shifts of two. They doubled up in rooms, so I got one pair ready for bed, and then the other.

Each night before bed, they flossed and brushed their teeth. Then I read them two stories, we said a prayer, and we sang two songs. Then I got out of the room so they could go to sleep.

—*Deborah Gilboa, MD, a mom of 14-, 12-, 10-, and 8-year-old sons, a family physician with Squirrel Hill Health Center, in Pittsburgh, PA, and a parenting speaker whose advice is found at AskDoctorG.com*

To help my husband and me get our sleep, we established a routine for *us.* I would nurse the baby at 7 pm, and then I'd go to sleep. My husband would wheel the baby in the bassinet into the living room.

### MomMy TIME: Give Yourself a Bath and Facial Before Bed

Your baby isn't the only one who can benefit from a bedtime routine. Indulging in a relaxing bath and taking time for self-care, such as giving yourself a facial or another home beauty treatment—all while the lights are low and avoiding the bright screens of electronics—will give you much-needed pampering time while helping prepare yourself for a restful night.

When the baby needed to eat at 10 or 11 pm, my husband would give her a bottle of pumped breast milk and change her diaper. Then he'd put the baby in the bassinet and go to sleep himself for the rest of the night.

I'd be "on" for the next feeding, but by then I had a stretch of five to six hours of sleep. That made all of the difference in the world to me. I could take on the night feedings without becoming too exhausted.

With this routine, our babies' early weeks weren't too taxing on my husband or me.

*—Marcela Dominguez, MD, a mom of a 13-year-old daughter and an 11-year-old son who has a private family medicine and wellness practice in Southern California, whose concierge medicine services are provided by Signature MD*

Sleep, not just for children but for doctors, is one of the favorite cocktail party conversations of emergency physicians. We dream about sleeping, and when the kids were small, we dreamed about *them* sleeping too.

For physicians—and also for babies—it's all about the schedule or lack thereof. Moms need to manipulate the schedule to maximize their own sleep time while still seeing their families at times when they are not exclusively sleeping.

Emergency docs don't work a fixed shift. Many physicians work a usual shift, such as days, and then they take call once a week. In emergency medicine, you rotate through five or six different shifts, and you might work all of them in a given week. You might not have the same three hours in bed two days in a row. This emphasizes why sleep comes hard for us, and it also emphasizes one of the fundamental principles for getting babies to sleep. It's really all about the schedule.

*—Rebecca Jeanmonod, MD, a mom of 12- and 8-year-old daughters and 11- and 8-year-old sons and a professor of emergency medicine and the associate residency program director for the emergency medicine residency at St. Luke's University Health Network, in Bethlehem, PA*

## Bathing

Babies might not be self-cleaning—like the cat!—but newborns really don't need baths every day. As long as you keep your baby's diaper area clean, he probably needs a bath only every three days.

However, many babies—and moms—love baths. Even super colicky babies are sometimes calmed by baths. If that's the case for your little one, giving him a bath every day is perfectly fine. You could skip the soap and just let your baby enjoy the soothing water. Your child might not be the happiest baby on the block, but at least he'll be the cleanest!

Baths are often part of bedtime routines, and for good reason. Baths are relaxing, and they help to set the stage for sleep. Because you need to focus 100 percent on your baby for safety's sake, baths are also great bonding, focused, one-on-one time.

⌒⁄◌

I think the very best sleep aid for my kids was their bath before bed. I think it was because the warm water seemed to relax them. Plus the excitement and energy spent during bathtime probably wore them out!

—*Leena S. Dev, MD, a mom of teenage boys and a general pediatrician, in Maryland.*

⌒⁄◌

My kids have bath time before bed nightly. It's a great routine for us and definitely helps my kids to feel warm and relaxed and cozy and to get ready for bed.

—*Sigrid Payne DaVeiga, MD*

⌒⁄◌

My husband and I always tried to make bath time part of a relaxing bedtime routine for our children. We used bath soaps with lavender, and then we massaged baby lotion on them after their baths to help them settle down. Lavender has always been an aromatherapy scent, which has been soothing for me. So I naturally thought it may also be helpful for my children..

—*Manpreet K. Gill, MD, a mom of a five-year-old daughter and a three-year-old son and a family practice physician with North Seminole Family Practice in Sanford, FL*

I gave my sons baths before bedtime. I think it was soothing for them. It's also a great time to bond with your baby. I tried to talk quietly with them to help them settle down for the night. All three of my sons did well with this simple nighttime routine.

—*Kristy Magee, MD, a mom of 15-, 12-, and 8-year-old sons and a family physician at North Seminole Family Practice and Sports Medicine, in Sanford, FL*

Our baby has mild eczema, so we wash her every other day to minimize drying of her skin. But she gets a little bit of supervised playtime in the tub every night to keep the routine. She knows that after messing herself after dinner, it's time to play in the water with her brother.

—*Edna Ma, MD, a mom of a 4-year-old son and an 18-month-old daughter, an anesthesiologist, and the founder of BareEASE pre-waxing numbing kit, in Los Angeles, CA*

Except in summertime when it was hot, I didn't give my babies a bath every night. Instead, I gave them baths a few times a week.

Because of this, I didn't make bathing part of the bedtime routine. You have to do things in the routine every single night. Consistency is the key to a successful bedtime routine.

—*Deborah Gilboa, MD*

## Massaging

Most babies love to be touched and massaged. Research suggests that infant massage can have health benefits. It might:

- Lessen crying—even colic
- Encourage one-on-one interaction between you and your baby
- Help your baby relax and even to fall asleep
- Reduce stress hormones
- Boost your baby's immune system
- Enhance your baby's motor skills
- Promote growth for premature babies

Certainly, massaging your baby will help *you* to relax and connect with him.

The best time to massage your baby is at least 45 minutes after he's eaten—less chance of him spitting up—and a bit before bedtime. If your baby cries or stiffens up, stop and try a massage another day. Then simply massage your baby in gentle, but firm strokes. No tickling! That's definitely not conducive to a bedtime routine!

We massage our children every night after bath time with organic almond or coconut oil.

—*Shilpa Amin-Shah, MD*

> **Touch comes before sight, before speech. It is the first language, and the last, and it always tells the truth.**
>
> —*Margaret Atwood, Canadian poet and novelist*

Our bedtime routine included a bath followed by a massage. A massage is ever so pleasant and relaxing, and it also stimulates a baby's developing brain.

—*Ayala Laufer-Cahana, MD*

❧

Offering gentle—or even more firm—touches on arms, legs, back, cheek, whatever your child likes, is also soothing during that getting-ready-for-bed time when they are too big to hold!

—*Katja Rowell, MD*

❧

I definitely used to massage my baby's little legs and feet before bedtime. It helped to soothe both of us. Even now, my son asks me to rub his feet when we are relaxing together at home.

—*Mona Gohara, MD, a mom of nine- and seven-year-old sons, a dermatologist in private practice, in Danbury, CT, and an associate clinical professor in the department of dermatology at Yale University*

## Mommy MD Guides–Recommended Product
### CeraVe Baby Moisturizing Lotion

CeraVe Baby Moisturizing Lotion is exceptionally soothing on my baby's skin. The texture of the cream is pleasant—not pasty or watery.

—Shilpa Amin-Shah, MD

The lotion moisturizes to help protect and maintain baby's delicate skin barrier for up to 24 hours. With three essential ceramides and vitamins, this moisturizing lotion also contains dimethicone, a skin protectant that helps temporarily relieve chafed, chapped, or cracked skin, leaving it feeling soft and moisturized. CeraVe Baby Moisturizing Lotion is hypoallergenic and fragrance-, paraben-, gluten-, sulfate-, and phthalate-free.

You can buy CeraVe Baby Moisturizing Lotion for $9.99 for an eight-ounce pump at drugstores, mass-market retailers, and specialty baby retailers nationwide. Visit **CeraVe.com** for more information.

My husband and I *loved* giving our babies massages. Sometimes it was before bed, usually right before or after bath time. We used to make up songs and teach the baby his body parts—arms, legs, face, back, tummy, hands, and feet.

—*Leena S. Dev, MD*

The routine and consistency of activities help set the stage for bedtime. I perform a post-bath baby massage each night after my daughter's bath. But now that she's 18 months old, and with her activity level, it's more of a wrestling and tickling match!

—*Edna Ma, MD*

The best way to soothe my baby was "her daddy." My poor husband used to lie next to her crib sometimes for an hour and just rub her back until she fell asleep. This happened for the first month or two and then recurred when she was teething. My husband definitely got tired, but never resentful. I'm married to one of the most loving, amazing men in the universe who's absolutely, completely devoted to "his girls." I think he took pride in the fact that he could do this for his baby.

—*Lisa M. Campanella-Coppo, MD, a mom of a six-year-old*
*daughter and an emergency department physician at Summit*
*Medical Group, in Livingston, NJ*

## Reading, Singing, Praying, and More

Here are the top 10 benefits to reading to your baby per Read-ToYourBaby.com:

- Promote listening skills
- Increase the number of vocabulary words heard
- Develop attention span and memory
- Help learn uncommon words
- Help learn to understand the meaning of words
- Learn concepts about print
- Learn to get information from illustrations
- Promote bonding and calmness for baby and mom
- Stimulate the imagination and senses
- Instill a love of books and learning

Read what you love! Your baby doesn't mind if you read comics or Cummings, cookbooks or Clarke. He just loves to hear the sound of your voice, and to feel the comfort of your arms.

∽⌒∾

My mother-in-law made audio tapes reading children's books. My kids loved listening to the stories, and they did so most nights.

—*Susan Besser, MD, a mom of six grown children, a grandmom of five, and a family physician at River Family Physicians, in Easton, MD*

∽⌒∾

We've read the same book to all three of our children—every day since they were born. I actually packed it in my hospital bag.

My husband and I feel that it's very important to establish a reading routine. We also love to send the baby to sleep with soothing words. I read *I Love You Through and Through.*

Now my 6-year-old son reads it to his 18-month-old sister at bedtime. It's so sweet!

—*Shilpa Amin-Shah, MD*

∽⌒∾

Because our new baby is only a month old, we have a new tradition of having his brother and sister read a few of our favorite bedtime stories to him before everyone settles down for the night. Our favorites are *The Hungry Caterpillar, Goodnight Gorilla, Goodnight Moon, Chicka Chicka Boom Boom,* and *Good Dog, Carl.*

This is a great way for all three of my kids to practice reading. My 10-year-old helps my 5-year-old sound out the words, and our baby sits in my lap listening closely to the story.

—*Sigrid Payne DaVeiga, MD*

∽⌒∾

I read to my babies from the time they were born. It was the last step in our nightly bedtime routine. I put reading last because that way my babies could look forward to all the pleasant things the end of the day brings, and they're all associated with going to bed.

—*Ayala Laufer-Cahana, MD*

> **A book is a dream that you hold in your hand.**
> —*Neil Gaiman, English author*

I loved singing to our daughter as part of her bedtime routine. We started doing this when she was a few months old, and we continued for years. I sang lullabies and songs that we learned in the music classes we took together.

I laughed one night when I heard my husband singing the theme song from *Gilligan's Island*. Singing TV theme songs, whatever, is fine!
—*Katja Rowell, MD*

Starting when my babies were around six months old, I would give them a sippy cup, and later a sports bottle, of water at bedtime. What's the downside, especially when they're still wearing diapers? It eliminates the "Mommy, I need a drink of water" excuse!
—*Deborah Gilboa, MD*

My kids have their own rooms, with a Jack-n-Jill bathroom in between. After I got them ready for nightime, I'd settle them each into bed. Then I'd open the doors between the bathroom, my husband would come upstairs, and we'd say prayers together. Then we'd shout "goodnight" with little nicknames. That is still the last step of our bedtime routine every night.
—*Lauren Hyman, MD, a mom of a 13-year-old daughter and an 11-year-old son and an ob-gyn at West Hills Hospital and Medical Center, in California*

My husband and I developed a bedtime routine that usually involves a story and some parental snuggling in bed for 5 or 10 minutes until our daughter relaxes and is ready to drift off.

She does occasionally get very clingy, especially when I am working too many days in a row. In fact, for the first time recently, she started insisting that I stay with her until she falls asleep and cries hysterically if I leave before she does. She wasn't falling asleep for almost 40 minutes past her bedtime.

There was a point when things were getting so bad that she'd come into my room two or three times a night and wake me up to come back to her room. During the moments of hysteria, I reassured her as best I could, but then when she was relaxed the next day, I explained to her that most parents who have more than one child can't snuggle their children like we do before bed and having us do that is a luxury. I also told her if she couldn't be a good girl and let us sleep and play by the rules of a time-limited snuggle, then we'd have to resort to just a kiss on the cheek at night and no snuggling so she wouldn't get so upset.

Of course, my daughter came back at me with "But, Mommy, don't you love to snuggle me?"

I said "Of course I do, and I would be so sad to not be able to do it anymore, but it's more important that we all get a good night's sleep so that we aren't tired for work and school."

I fear I sound like a horrible mother for doing this, but my daughter got the message, and for now we are back to a 10-minute bedtime snuggle until she is drowsy, and then off we go.

—*Lisa M. Campanella-Coppo, MD*

The most difficult sleep challenge for my babies was getting them to sleep when there was a change in routine. Sometimes, such as if I worked late, it was simply impossible to stick to the routine, in which case I would try to do at least two or three things that were part of the routine. If the routine included bathing, drying off, applying lotion, rocking, and feeding, followed by more rocking with a silky and a pacifier, I might make sure I put on lotion if we couldn't have a bath or make sure there was still the familiar silky and a bit of rocking right before going to bed.

—*Kathryn Boling, MD, a mom of two grown daughters, a grandmom of two, and a family medicine physician with Mercy Medical Center, in Baltimore, MD*

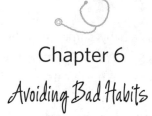

# Chapter 6
## Avoiding Bad Habits

Sleep challenges among new moms are so common there's actually a name for it: postnatal insomnia. A National Sleep Foundation poll discovered that 74 percent of stay-at-home moms had insomnia. (We worry about the other 26 percent. Perhaps they were too sleep deprived to understand the question.)

Motherhood can bring such intense sleep challenges and sleep deprivation that you might wonder: Is it possible to die from being this tired? Extreme sleep deprivation can cause one to do some pretty crazy things to try to get to sleep. Sleep aides and alcohol might seem like easy answers and quick fixes. But they come with side effects.

Rather than trading one problem (insomnia) for a worse one (bad habits or even addictions), establish healthier habits instead. For example, taking a walk, doing yoga, or listening to meditation can help you unwind, relax, and sleep better —and they don't come with warning labels.

## JUSTIFICATION FOR A CELEBRATION
Any time your baby goes to sleep sans nursing is a reason to celebrate.

> **I love sleep. My life has the tendency
> to fall apart when I'm awake, you know?**
> —*Ernest Hemingway*

## Rocking or Swinging the Baby to Sleep

"Rock-a-Bye Baby"—how could such a sweet song be wrong?

∼

When my daughter was a baby, sometimes she really gave us a hard time about going to sleep. We had a motorized rocking swing she would sleep in when we were desperate, especially for naptime. We would put it on the fastest speed. To this day, I still can't believe we didn't make baby milk shakes come back up after her meals, but the rocking swing was a godsend.

> —Lisa M. Campanella-Coppo, MD, a mom of a six-year-old daughter and an emergency department physician at Summit Medical Group, in Livingston, NJ

**BABY SLEEP PRO TIP: Create Positive Sleep Associations**

One of the keys to lengthening night sleep is helping your baby learn to self-soothe by creating positive sleep associations. These are present at bedtime and when your child wakes in the middle of the night; therefore, your child can fall back to sleep independently. Negative sleep associations are the root of many children's night wakings and sleep issues. Whatever it takes to get your child to sleep in the first place will need to happen again when he wakes in the middle of the night. Focus on replacing negative sleep associations with positive ones, so your baby can fall asleep independently.

| POSITIVE SLEEP ASSOCIATIONS | NEGATIVE SLEEP ASSOCIATIONS |
| --- | --- |
| Sleeping in a certain way. | Nursing or bottle to sleep. |
| Sleeping with a favorite object, stuffed animal, or lovey. | Holding, rocking, or bouncing to sleep. |
| Using white noise or a fan continuously for sleep. | Car rides, swing, or other motion to sleep. |
| Sleeping in the dark with the door open or closed. | Patting, singing, or walking to sleep. |

> —Rebecca Kempton, MD

> **A mother's arms are made of tenderness, and children sleep soundly in them.**
>
> *—Victor Hugo, poet*

I never rocked my babies to sleep. Our nighttime routine always included a bath—or at least a good wipe down—and nursing in a rocking chair. I never let them fall asleep while being rocked, though! I put my babies into their cribs before they fell asleep.

Sure, they cried. I would go in and check on them and give them a bit of reassurance, but then I would leave again. Sometimes I had to repeat that cycle. But as a result, my kids both slept through the night by the time they were about four months old.

*—Antoinette Cheney, DO, a mom of a 12-year-old son and an 11-year-old daughter, and a family physician with Rocky Vista University College of Osteopathic Medicine, in Parker, CO*

If I could give just one piece of advice for new parents, this is what it would be: Get your baby into the habit of falling asleep *by himself, in his own bed.* You do not want your baby's sleep to depend on your presence.

Although it doesn't seem apparent at first, and it's delightful to have your baby fall asleep in your arms, the secret to keeping your life balanced is to have a routine that works for the entire family. The novelty of rocking a baby to sleep, or walking with him up and down the stairs until he finally snoozes (only to wake up once you put him down), quickly wears off. Evenings wasted waiting for a little time off are exhausting.

A baby's ability to calm himself independently—and to feel secure when you're not in the room—is important for his development, and for your sanity.

*—Ayala Laufer-Cahana, MD, a mom of 20- and 18-year-old sons and a 17-year-old daughter, a pediatrician, artist, entrepreneur, and founder of Herbal Water Inc. and DrAyala.com, in greater Philadelphia, PA*

Every generation seems to be sharply focused on a particular aspect of infancy. In the early part of the 20th century, there was tremendous emphasis on a baby's bowel movements and the importance of enforcing a strictly structured schedule with laxatives and enemas. Yet all of this careful frenzy about bowel movements seems to have entirely disappeared. Likewise, somewhat later in mid-century, there was an enormous focus on "modern" feedings of infants with "scientific" formulas and carefully regimented attention to the clock. This approach too seems to have passed into oblivion, with a more recent resurgence of breastfeeding and on-demand feeding among mothers over the past 50 years.

But now, the current crop of infants seems to be in need of "training" in order to sleep. An anthropologist might have fun analyzing these fads, but most mothers all over the world would probably find these developments quite puzzling.

There are probably sensible hints regarding sleep that could be developed by experts using current research methods—recommendations based on genuine evidence. At the moment, however, we are still awaiting real wisdom. When it comes, wisdom will probably arrive in a form that involves a combination of empathic parental awareness of the baby's own cues and a gentle attempt to move the baby's sleep pattern in the right direction.

Along these lines, it seems to be helpful to put newborns and small infants into their beds to sleep when they are awake, right from

## Mommy MD Guides–Recommended Product
### Boppy Head Support
Keep your newborn's head in a comfortable position when she's in her bouncy seat, stroller, or swing with this head support. It fits babies from preemies up to 12 months. You can buy it for $24 at Pottery Barn Kids. For more information or to order, visit **POTTERY-BARNKIDS.COM.**

the start. The attempt to have the baby fall asleep in your arms or at the breast, and then to carefully transfer the snoozing infant to bed without waking the baby is a well-intentioned approach, but it seems to make for problems later on. Establishing the pattern that babies are put down to sleep when they are sleepy but still awake seems to work best; that way, the baby gets into the routine of tolerating a bit of wakefulness before slumber. Parents who want to make sure that the baby is asleep before placing the child into the crib may be encouraging the baby to expect this treatment indefinitely. Then the baby is outraged by being put to bed while still awake.

Subtly molding the child's experiences so that the child gradually expects and accepts more mature patterns of living is thus not a "training" program but an overall aspect of the parental relationship with the child. The child is not an employee or trainee or student. The parent is alert to the child's feelings and the child's situation and works with these to move things gradually in a forward direction. This is an approach that characterizes many facets of parenting in addition to sleep.

—*Elizabeth Berger, MD, a mom of two grown children, a child psychiatrist, and the author of* Raising Kids with Character, *in New York City*

❧

I really felt that because I was a woman, a pediatrician, and someone who had surrounded herself with children growing up (babysitting, etc.), I would know everything there was to know about raising a baby. Boy, was I wrong!

When my son was a newborn, he would only sleep while being held, wouldn't sleep in a swing for very long, would fuss if I was lying next to him, would fuss if I *didn't* lie next to him, would be comforted while being rocked but then the rocking was too much, liked being held but only when I was standing. In short, he would cry no matter what I did.

I did research and talked with anyone who would give me any information. I read every sleep book and journal out there. Because there was so much conflicting information (feed on demand versus feed on a schedule, co-sleep versus don't co-sleep, hold baby to sleep versus always put him in a crib), it was overwhelming, to say the least.

Plus, it was tricky figuring out when he was hungry versus sleepy. It all seemed to overlap in the beginning days. I felt like I didn't know my own child.

Once I took a deep breath and trusted my gut (and leaning on the stuff I learned from the books), I started relaxing and things started improving. I noticed that my baby responded to my mood and behavior. When I was anxious, my child was fussy. When I was relaxed, my child was relaxed.

When I figured out my baby's cues and this ebb and flow with myself, a lot of things fell into place. He became a better feeder, was in a better mood, and slept better as well. Having the support of my husband was also crucial in this process.

My advice in this matter is to do what you have to do in the first three months. It's all about survival. After you have gotten to know your baby, and your baby has gotten to know you, you can work on establishing good rules and not feeding or rocking your baby to sleep.

—*Nilong Parikh Vyas, MD, MPH, a mom of seven- and five-year-old sons and the founder and owner of Sleepless in NOLA sleep consulting, in New Orleans, LA*

## Nursing the Baby to Sleep

Sleepy baby plus drowsy mama often equals both of you falling asleep while nursing. Whether this is a problem or not is a matter of degrees! Newborns falling asleep while nursing occasionally is lovely. Older babies crying for you to come nurse them to sleep 11 times a night is not!

After that honeymoon at the hospital, my first son seemed to never sleep upon arriving home—despite near perfect conditions! Although I had read every sleep book I could get my hands on, apparently he didn't read the same ones.

My main challenge was getting him to sleep for any length of time day or night without needing me in some capacity—nursing, rocking, bouncing, pacing, changing. I was sleep deprived, and so was he. I was also desperate for a lifeline, someone to help me figure out the sleep thing. Nine months in, I decided to let my son cry for one night out of pure desperation, and amazingly, after 273 days of interrupted sleep, he slept!

*—Rebecca Kempton, MD, a mom of eight- and six-year-old sons and a three-year-old-daughter and an infant and toddler sleep specialist, in Chicago, IL*

∽

From the newborn period until a baby is about four months old, it is absolutely okay to nurse a baby to sleep. I did! Nursing is soothing to them.

By the time a baby is four to six months old, she needs to start learning to soothe herself. I didn't learn this in medical school; I learned it as a parent.

Once my babies were about four months old and weighed 15 pounds, I started the process of transitioning them to falling asleep in their cribs. At 15 pounds, babies no longer nutritionally need milk in the night.

I would hold my baby until she got drowsy. Then I would gently place her in her crib—awake. If she fell asleep, great! If she fussed, I got her up. I repeated this process until she fell asleep on her own. Sometimes I would stand next to her crib with my hand on her back to soothe her.

## Give Up the Night Cap

It can be tempting to turn to a glass of wine to help get to sleep faster, but drinking before bed is a bad habit that's worth kicking. Yes, a drink at bedtime may help you fall asleep, but alcohol disturbs your sleep cycles for the entire night, causing you to go through only one or two sleep cycles rather than the usual six or seven that help you feel well-rested.

If you drink, do it at least two hours before bed for every glass of wine or three hours before bed for every glass of beer to allow your body to process the alcohol before sleeping.

> **The woods are lovely, dark and deep. But I have promises to keep, and miles to go before I sleep.**
>
> —*Robert Frost*

It took a few days, and great consistency, but after that my babies fell asleep on their own in their cribs. It helps to understand that it can take up to 20 minutes for a drowsy infant to fall asleep.

> —*Eva Mayer, MD, a mom of a 12-year-old daughter and an 11-year-old son, an associate professor of pediatrics at Temple University, and a pediatrician with St. Luke's Hospital Coopersburg Pediatrics, in Pennsylvania*

⁓

It's okay for newborns to fall asleep on the breast. If this is still happening when the baby is two to six months old, however, this is not good.

Any bad habit can be broken. At four to six months of age, babies develop mature sleep cycles. They learn to self-soothe when they partially awaken during the night, like all people do. Adults naturally partially awaken during the night to ensure safety—for example, to make sure that there's no fire—and when reassured, they instantly go back to sleep.

Babies are just learning how to do this. At first, they wake up and wonder, *Hey, where is everyone and my nipple?* This is the point when they can be trained to self-soothe—without the breast or even a pacifier. At about six months, three nights of sleep training will help the child sleep through the night, as long as the baby weighs more than 15 pounds and is free of health issues.

> —*Hana R. Solomon, MD, a mom of four grown biological children, two grown "spiritually adopted" children, a grandmom of eight, a pediatrician, the president of BeWell Health, LLC, the inventor of Dr. Hana's Nasopure nose wash for children, and the author of* Clearing the Air One Nose at a Time: Caring for Your Personal Filter, *in Columbia, MO*

## RALLIE'S TIP

*I loved nursing each of my babies. I had my middle son when I was in my second year of medical residency. When I came home from a long day of working at the hospital, I couldn't wait to scoop up my baby and nurse him. It was our special snuggling and bonding time. I wanted to hold him as long as I could before bedtime, because I knew I'd have to get up early for work the next day.*

*I made the serious mistake of allowing my son to nurse until he fell asleep most evenings. Sometimes I dozed off right along with him.*

*Before I knew it, I had created a demanding little monster. My son wouldn't even think about going to sleep at night unless he was in my arms and nursing. He might be sound asleep, but whenever I tried to remove him from my breast and put him in his crib for the night, he would instantly be wide awake and start to wail. It wasn't his fault; I had inadvertently conditioned him to associate nursing with falling asleep.*

*It took a long time and a lot of crying and missed sleep to reverse this pattern, but it was a very good lesson for me. When my youngest son was born, I was completing my final year of residency. I still cuddled and nursed him when I came home from work in the evenings, but I made sure that we both stayed awake.*

*As soon as my son had his fill, I ended his nursing session and put him in his crib to go to sleep. We still got to snuggle and bond, and we both slept better!*

### Take the Baby for a Walk

Sun exposure can have a positive impact on your circadian rhythms, which means taking a morning walk in the sunshine will help you and your baby sleep better at night. One 2014 study of workers found that those exposed to sunlight during the day slept more hours at night. You can do the same by getting out the stroller, strapping your baby in, and heading out for a walk while giving yourself a break from your other mommy duties.

# Chapter 7

# Napping

"Sleep when your baby sleeps." Like so many things in parenting, it sounds so simple, so logical—yet so impossible, so unattainable.

When you get your baby to nap, you suddenly feel pulled in 18 directions at once: Do you fold the laundry that's spilling out of the clothes dryer? Or do you catch up with long-lost friends on Facebook? Do you try to return your mother-in-law's phone call? Or do you catch up on DVR'd episodes of Sister Wives?

Once your little one closes his eyes for a nap, you know nap time will fly by in what feels like the blink of an eye. It's tempting to make nap time productive. But the irony is: The most productive thing you could probably do is take a nap yourself!

## JUSTIFICATION FOR A CELEBRATION
You got to take a nap today too!

> **A day without a nap**
> **is like a cupcake without frosting.**
> *—Terri Guillemets,*
> *quotation anthologist*

## Napping Schedules

Clocks and time, light and darkness don't have much effect on newborn babies' sleep. Newborns alternate between sleeping and eating—round the clock. As your baby gets older, his sleeping and waking become more regular and predictable.

At around four months old, most babies take one morning and one afternoon nap. If you're really lucky, your baby might also take a second, late afternoon nap. (Congratulations! You won the naptime lottery!)

It's also around four months old that babies start to form sleep associations. That means they understand the link between "hey, this is my crib" and "hey, this is where I sleep!" We hope anyway. Or your baby might get the link between "hey, this is my mom's breast" and "hey, this is what I *need* to fall asleep!" This is why it's a good idea to put your baby in his crib or bassinet for at least one nap to get him used to the idea of crib=sleep.

*In the beginning, my babies both took three naps a day, following mealtimes. When my babies were about eight months old, they went down to two naps.*

> —*Edna Ma, MD, a mom of a 4-year-old son and an 18-month-old daughter, an anesthesiologist, and the founder of BareEASE pre-waxing numbing kit, in Los Angeles, CA*

*At first, babies are only awake for 4 hours in a 24-hour period. As my babies got older, I tried to structure their naps as much as possible. They would nap for one to two hours in the morning and one to two hours in the afternoon.*

*When it's time for my baby's nap, I put on music in her room, put her in her crib, and leave. This way, she knows it's naptime. I think she thinks, I'm in my crib. The music's on. It must be naptime! My baby usually falls asleep immediately.*

> —*Aline T. Tanios Keyrouz, MD, a mom of 13- and 7-year-old and 9-month-old daughters and an 11-year-son and an assistant professor of pediatrics at St. Louis University, in Missouri*

I never let my babies fall asleep after feedings during the day. The routine was eat, awake time, and then put them down in the crib in their own room for a nap. I believe that this schedule taught them to fall asleep without outside influence.

My naptimes were pretty rigid, within a half hour or so. I always planned my day around that. It was inconvenient, but it was a necessity for me.

*—Antoinette Cheney, DO, a mom of a 12-year-old son and an 11-year-old daughter, and a family physician with Rocky Vista University College of Osteopathic Medicine, in Parker, CO*

In general, we kept very close to our routine, which worked well for our family. We had a kiddo who ate well, slept well, and was content. We found that the routine seemed to be a big part of that. Of course, then we didn't have as many outings in the evenings, and we planned to be home for naptimes. That worked for us.

Some families choose to be more adventurous or spontaneous, and that's a fine choice as well, but it may make sleep more challenging. It's all a trade-off.

With our family, a pretty regular schedule from day to day was a key to our baby's mood. Her rhythm became pretty predictable—until she started to drop her naps!

*—Katja Rowell, MD, a mom of a 10-year-old daughter, a family practice physician, and the author of* Helping Your Child with Extreme Picky Eating and Love Me, Feed Me *at TheFeedingDoctor.com, in St. Paul, MN*

My firstborn never napped consistently, and even now as a five year old, she still has trouble settling down to sleep. When she was only 10 months old, she stopped taking her morning nap at home, but she would still nap between 12 and 2 pm in day care. Sometimes we would have to drive her around the block to help her nap.

On the other hand, my youngest has always slept well. During his first year, he took at least two or three naps a day, and he was relatively easy to put down to sleep. Now that he's three years old, he can sometimes go without a nap at home, but he usually naps between 12 and 2 pm at school. Even at home, he'll nap from 1 to 3 pm on weekends.

—*Manpreet K. Gill, MD, a mom of a five-year-old daughter and a three-year-old son and a family practice physician with North Seminole Family Practice, in Sanford, FL*

❧

When my new baby and I came home from the hospital, I tried to follow the familiar advice of "nap when your baby naps." This is easier said than done, especially if you have older children.

Many people will give you this advice. Initially, it will not make sense because you have so much to do, and you'll want to do it when the baby naps. But the more experienced you become as a mom, the more you will realize the wisdom in sleeping while your baby sleeps. Because your baby needs to get up every two to three hours at night to eat, you won't be getting good quality sleep at night. If you don't nap when your baby naps, you will end up with sleep deprivation and exhaustion. This creates a vicious cycle: You get tired. Your milk production decreases. You might already be struggling with postpartum depression, and sleep deprivation will make that worse. This will make you feel even more tired.

## Mommy MD Guides-Recommended Product
### Graco Pack 'n Play Playard Everest

If you prefer a playard with all the bells and whistles, check out Graco's Pack 'n Play Playard Everest. In addition to the playard and removable infant bassinet, it also comes with a portable lounger with two speeds of vibration and a toy bar. It also includes a changing table and ample space to organize diapers and wipes. The lounger and changer can be used with babies up to 30 pounds.

The playard comes in two patterns: a black, gray, and red design and another with gray tones and light teal blue. It sells for $319.99 from Graco's website, **GRACOBABY.COM.**

It's important to nap, and it's important to delegate. Ask for help with cooking, cleaning, and feeding the baby. Your main goals for the first few weeks of motherhood are to maintain your sanity and to sleep.

—*Aline T. Tanios Keyrouz, MD*

✐

Sleep is about schedule. Once my babies were on anything resembling a schedule, we followed it. For all four of my babies, about two hours after they had breakfast, we put them down for a nap even if they didn't look tired. If you wait until your baby looks tired to put him down for a nap, it's too late. The fussing wakes babies up and makes it hard for them to relax and settle down.

So two hours after breakfast, whether our babies thought they needed a nap or not, we put them down to sleep. Almost invariably, they went to sleep and took a morning nap.

Then they'd get up again, be awake for a bit, and about two hours after they ate their lunches, we'd put them down again. This schedule worked well right through toddlerhood.

Even when our kids no longer needed that morning nap every day, it gave them the opportunity to have quiet time.

—*Rebecca Jeanmonod, MD, a mom of 12- and 8-year-old daughters and 11- and 8-year-old sons and a professor of emergency medicine and the associate residency program director for the emergency medicine residency at St. Luke's University Health Network, in Bethlehem, PA*

## Time Your Best Nap

Experts say the best time to nap is mid-afternoon because it's less likely to affect your sleep at night, so try to lie down around 2 pm.

You can use a sleep app on your phone that includes a nap setting. Or download a power nap app that will wake you after 20 to 30 minutes.

Timing is, as they say, everything!

> **Learn from yesterday, live for today,**
> **look to tomorrow, rest this afternoon.**
>
> —*Charles M. Schulz,*
> **Charlie Brown's Little Book of Wisdom**

## Napping Location

As you careen through your new-mom days, with barely time to use the bathroom let alone plan out your day, it might be tempting to put your baby down for a nap "in place," such as on a couch or chair, or on *you* as you fall asleep on a couch or chair. Don't! These are not safe napping locations.

Just as you do at bedtime, put your baby to nap in his crib or bassinet, on his back, without any toys, bumpers, or blankets. This is best for your baby, and it's also best for you! Once your baby is safe in his crib or bassinet, you can go do something productive, relaxing, or better yet, fun!

My first baby was cranky and refluxy. I didn't worry about where he napped; I was just happy that he was napping at all. My baby napped a lot on me! He also napped in the Pack 'n Play or in a bouncy seat. I had a really cool mini bassinet that he liked.

My second baby fell asleep for his naps much more quickly in the bassinet or crib.

—*Heather Orman-Lubell, MD, a mom of 15- and 11-year-old*
*sons and a pediatrician at St. Chris Care at Yardley Pediatrics, in*
*Pennsylvania*

When my baby first came home from the hospital, we had a Pack 'n Play with a bassinet insert downstairs that she would nap in. If needed, I tried to take a shower during her naps. I would put her down in her crib upstairs.

—*Jeannette Gonzalez Simon, DO, a mom of seven- and five-*
*year-old daughters and a pediatric gastroenterologist in Verona, NJ*

When my twins first came home from the hospital, we put them down for naps based upon their needs. In time, we developed more of a set schedule. They would take about three naps. two in the morning, and one in the afternoon. Initially they napped in two bassinets in our living room. Later, we transitioned naps to their bedroom, which was quiet and darker.

—*Sonal R. Patel, MD, a mom of four-year-old twin daughters and a physician who specializes in pediatric/adult allergy and immunology with Adventist Health Physicians Network, in Los Angeles, CA*

With my first babies, it was easier to have them on a set nap schedule and have them nap at home in their cribs. With my new baby, I also have older kids, who have busy schedules of their own. We're often on the go, and our schedule is often messed up. Because of this, my baby is accustomed to sleeping anywhere, such as in her car seat or stroller.

I think this is a good thing. I've heard people say, "My kids won't sleep in the car." I think, *If you have to take a 10-hour road trip, what are you going to do?* It's best if kids have some flexibility.

—*Aline T. Tanios Keyrouz, MD*

## Mommy MD Guides-Recommended Product
### C Sleep

Sometimes a product comes along that makes you think: *Wow, what did we do before this?* The C Sleep by GE is a Bluetooth-enabled light bulb that's designed to help get you ready for sleep at night and support your body's natural sleep/wake cycle during the day.

The C Sleep bulb is specially designed for bedrooms. It features three settings: a cool, vibrant light that helps get you going in the morning, a standard daytime light, and a warm light that doesn't impede melatonin production before bed and supports circadian rhythms.

The C Sleep is available at Target in a 2-pack for around $50 and in a single pack at Lowe's for around $25. Visit **www.cbyge .com**, **Lowes.com** or **Target.com** for more information.

When our kids first came home from the hospital, they napped in a bassinet or crib in their rooms as much as possible. We wanted them to get used to sleeping at regular intervals in a regular place. The more consistently we followed the routine, the faster they learned it.

Our twins were our last pregnancy, and I didn't want them hurting the schedules of my older children, one of whom was two and the other who had just turned four. The twins napped in car seats in opposite corners of our family room. This worked well because when one would cry, I could tell by which direction the sound came from which infant was hungry or restless.

This was incredibly important at night when the twins were feeding on demand. It's unbelievable how many times one would cry and then stop just as I'd open my eyes. If I didn't have them sleeping apart, I wouldn't have known which one had cried.

I let them sleep in their car seats early on, even at night. This was because they had to share rooms with their two- and four-year-old siblings. I didn't want all four to have disrupted sleep. So for the first several months, they slept in their car seats, until we moved our older son and daughter into a single room and put the twins, also a boy and a girl, in another room together. We kept them split like that until the twins were four years old because the small children had one schedule, and the older children had a different one.

—*Rebecca Jeanmonod, MD*

## Recognizing Signs of Drowsiness

Veteran moms will tell you to watch your baby for signs of drowsiness. They might be more subtle than signs of *moms'* drowsiness, which include:

- Calling your child by the wrong kid's name
- Calling your child by the cat's name
- Putting the car keys in the fridge
- Driving for four blocks before realizing you're headed in the wrong direction
- Staring at your laptop screen trying to figure out what you're supposed to be doing

- Walking into a room and forgetting what you went in for
- Falling asleep six seconds into your favorite TV show
- Finally crawling into bed, where you lie awake for hours

I could always tell that my daughters were tired when they started rubbing their eyes and faces with their hands or when they rubbed their faces against my chest.

—*Jeannette Gonzalez Simon, DO*

All three of my children have been pretty different sleepers. What worked for one baby did not necessarily work for the others.

I am a big believer in reading children's signals. I watched my babies for signs that they were tired and then got them into bed.

**BABY SLEEP PRO TIP:** Understand Sleepy Cues

Your baby's signs of tiredness, or sleepy cues, are important for you to recognize early on. Understanding your baby's sleep cues will help you know when to put your baby to sleep before she gets overtired, which is a key to successful sleep!

What do sleepy cues look like? All babies are different, so observe your baby closely to learn what signs he gives you when he is tired.

**Here are some common sleep cues:**
- Decreased activity and slowing movement
- Zoning out; less engaged
- Less vocal, calmer
- Batting at ears; pulling hair
- Drooping eyelids; glazed eyes
- Rubbing eyes

Important: Yawning and fussiness are usually indicative of being overtired!

—*Rebecca Kempton, MD*

*—Sigrid Payne DaVeiga, MD, a mom of 10-year-old and 1-month-old sons and a 5-year-old daughter and a pediatric allergist with the Children's Hospital of Philadelphia, in Pennsylvania*

∽

My husband and I knew our baby was tired if she began to hold her lovey and rub her eyes with it. She would also get less active and more cuddly.

Some kiddos are very clear with their signs; others not so much. I think we got pretty lucky with our daughter. Her signs of drowsiness were easy to spot.

*—Katja Rowell, MD*

∽

Day to day, I didn't look for my children to get drowsy. My goal was to have them in bed *before* they knew they were tired and have them asleep before they knew it too.

Occasionally, when we were out during their naptime, running errands, or on a vacation, my babies would get tired. This mostly looked like fussing, irritability, rubbing their faces, or arching their backs. Once my babies got to that point, it was much harder to get them to sleep. If they got to that point, they needed to be rocked, bounced, soothed, and helped to get to their "happy places" and sleep.

I always preferred keeping my babies on their schedules because it taught them to soothe themselves to sleep.

*—Rebecca Jeanmonod, MD*

### Mommy Time: Taking a Nap

Recharging with a 20- to 30-minute nap makes a happier and more alert mommy. Most likely, you'll be napping when your child is sleeping in the afternoon, which is good timing because an afternoon nap shouldn't interfere with your ability to go to sleep at night.

You can help yourself fall asleep by choosing the same time to lie down every day and by creating an environment that will lead to sleep, which means setting a comfortable temperature and making your room as dark as possible.

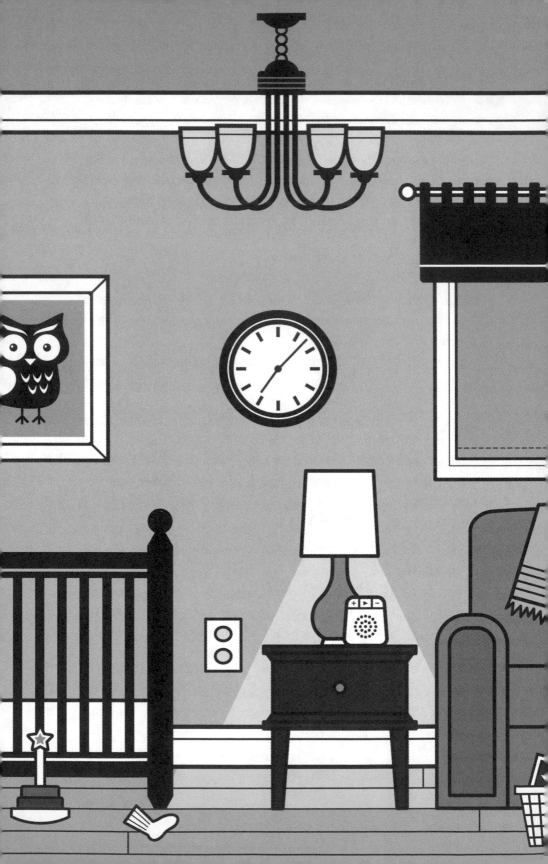

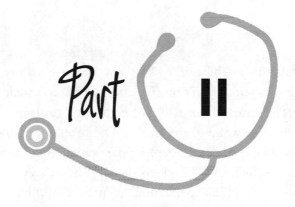

# Part II

## BABIES: 1 MONTH TO 1 YEAR

# Chapter 8
## Dealing with Nighttime Wakings

We all wake up in the night. The key is, once you've assured yourself that the house isn't on fire and you haven't slept through your 8 am meeting, you usually fall right back to sleep.

Babies, too, wake in the night. The problem is, they don't know how to fall back to sleep. In particular, they don't know how to soothe themselves back to sleep. When parents call their kids "good" or "bad" sleepers, more accurate might be "good" or "bad" soothers. If your baby doesn't know how to soothe herself back to sleep, naturally she calls out to the one person she knows will help—you.

Interestingly, studies have found an association between babies with "difficult" temperaments and problem sleep. These "difficult" babies are less likely to be able to soothe themselves. As babies learn to soothe themselves, they sleep better, and longer, through the night. The question is: How can you teach your baby to soothe herself, and can you do it by tonight?

### JUSTIFICATION FOR A CELEBRATION
Treat yourself to a special coffee or tea to celebrate when neither your baby—nor you!—woke for a midnight meal.

> **If we're not meant to have a midnight snack,**
> **why is there a light in the fridge?**
>
> **—Anonymous**

## Waking to Feed

By the time infants are around six months old, they are physically capable of sleeping through the night. But of course that doesn't mean they *do*!

When babies wake at night to eat, it's called "night feedings." After six months, these feedings are less about actually being hungry, and more about habit or about needing help to go back to sleep. Just like you don't need a Dagwood sandwich at 2 am to fall back to sleep, your baby doesn't really need a nighttime nursing either.

When your baby is between four months and one year old, it's important to establish healthy sleep habits because your baby's sleep patterns become more adult-like. Of course, this doesn't happen overnight! This is sometimes called "night weaning." Probably the most painless way for you—and your baby—is to slowly drop off one night feeding every few nights.

❧

My children only woke to breastfeed in their first few months. Initially for both of my children, in the first few weeks of life, I was nursing every two to four hours during the day and every four hours at night. I found that each baby is different. My son could sleep for five to six hour stretches at night within the first month of age on his own, without changing anything in our routine.

—*Manpreet K. Gill, MD, a mom of a five-year-old daughter and a three-year-old son and a family practice physician with North Seminole Family Practice, in Sanford, FL*

### ♥ Get Back to Sleep

If you wake up in the middle of the night for longer than 20 minutes, get out of bed and do something that will help you relax, recommends the National Institutes of Health. Once you feel sleepy again, get back into bed. Taking this step takes away the anxiety of lying in bed not being able to sleep, which can make sleep even more elusive.

Neither of my children slept through the night for ages—until they were 14 months old! My son woke nightly to feed until he was 10 months old. My daughter had this habit until about eight months, at which time we did sleep training to preserve our sanity!

—*Edna Ma, MD, a mom of a 4-year-old son and an 18-month-old daughter, an anesthesiologist, and the founder of BareEASE pre-waxing numbing kit, in Los Angeles, CA*

The first two months of my babies' lives were hard. When they were infants and they woke in the night, I only woke up long enough to find out if they were hungry. If they were hungry, I fed them.

If they weren't hungry, my husband helped. My younger son liked to be bounced. My husband would literally stand on the bed and bounce the baby up and down. I learned to sleep right through it.

—*Sharon Boyce, MD, a mom of seven- and five-year-old sons and a family physician with Oaklawn Medical Group, in Albion and Bellevue, MI*

### Sleep When Your Baby Sleeps

Everyone from your mother to strangers who coo at your baby in the supermarket is probably giving you the sage advice to sleep when your baby sleeps during those months that she's still waking you in the middle of the night. There's good reason for this advice. A 2014 study on sleepiness among new mothers found that half of the mothers studied were still excessively sleepy when their babies were 18 weeks old.

How do you catch some zzz's in the middle of the day during your baby's catnaps? Start by turning off your phone and then turn your back on household chores, which can wait until your baby is up again. Then close the blinds, keep the temperature at a comfortable level, and lie down for a rest.

At night, my baby would fall asleep easily. For her first six weeks, even if she was in a deep sleep, I woke her every three hours to eat. I set an alarm so I would wake up. Babies' blood sugar can drop too low if they go too long without eating.

When my baby was six weeks old and weighed about 12 pounds, I stopped waking her to eat. By then I accepted—even *expected*—that she could sleep through the night.

—*Aline T. Tanios Keyrouz, MD, a mom of 13- and 7-year-old and 9-month-old daughters and an 11-year-son and an assistant professor of pediatrics at St. Louis University, in Missouri*

∽

If our baby woke up, we addressed her needs and fed her or changed her diaper, but she slept through the night almost from the first day. For those of you who would like to hate me, don't worry, we were lucky for about six months, but then she woke us up three times a night once she started teething!

—*Lisa M. Campanella-Coppo, MD, a mom of a six-year-old daughter and an emergency department physician at Summit Medical Group, in Livingston, NJ*

## Waking to Be Changed

In a baby's first few months of life, she pees about 20 times in a 24-hour period. Certainly, you don't change her diaper each time even during the day, let alone at night. That would be expensive!

It's definitely not necessary to wake a sleeping baby to change her. (We advocate waking a sleeping baby, well, practically never.) If your baby wakes for another reason, and you notice her diaper needs to be changed, perhaps because her pjs are wet, turn on as little light and make as little noise as possible. Be quick, but gentle, changing her so as not to wake her any more then necessary. And hopefully your baby—and you—can go back to sleep quickly.

∽

A funny thing about my kids is how different they have been about having a wet diaper. My daughter would cry when she had a wet

> ### How Much Sleep Does a Baby Need?
> Once your baby is four months old or older, she should get somewhere between 12 to 15 hours of sleep a day, keeping in mind that a few hours more or a few hours less is nothing to be concerned about. However, if your baby is sleeping more than 16 hours a day or less than 10 hours a day, it could indicate a problem that would require a talk with your pediatrician.

diaper, and after we changed her diaper, she would feel better and fall back asleep restfully. My one-month-old son cries any time we try to change his diaper, so we try to not disturb him while he is sleeping so that he can get good rest.

—*Sigrid Payne DaVeiga, MD, a mom of 10-year-old and 1-month-old sons and a 5-year-old daughter and a pediatric allergist with the Children's Hospital of Philadelphia, in Pennsylvania*

We only changed our babies diapers if they woke and we noticed their diapers were wet. Personally, having lived in wet clothes for 33 days on an island during the taping of the *Survivor* TV show, it was a priority for me to change my babies out of any wet clothes or diapers immediately. Wet clothes and diapers are uncomfortable, and they can also cool a child's body temperature. And children are not developed enough to auto-regulate their temperature.

—*Edna Ma, MD*

When my babies were eight or nine months old, both of them would wake during the night when they were wet, soaking through their clothes. We would quickly try to change them and get them back to sleep.

We tried using different diapers and then overnight diapers. With my second child, I started layering crib sheets, with waterproof liners in between, which made it easier to quickly change the bedding.

—*Manpreet K. Gill, MD*

If I heard my babies make a noise in the middle of the night, I would stand by the door and peek in to make sure they were okay. I had a five-minute rule before intervening. Most of the time, babies will work through things and fall back to sleep. My husband and I wanted our babies to learn how to do this on their own.

If the crying continued, I would go to the crib, reach over the top of the crib, and help my baby find her finger or thumb. I'd hold it in her mouth for a little bit. That would usually comfort her enough to fall back to sleep.

—*Marcela Dominguez, MD, a mom of a 13-year-old daughter and an 11-year-old son who has a private family medicine and wellness practice in Southern California, whose concierge medicine services are provided by Signature MD*

## Mommy MD Guides–Recommended Product
### Triple Paste

My daughter used to be very prone to diaper rash. I discovered Triple Paste, and that's now my go-to cream. I put Triple Paste on my babies every night before putting on the overnight diaper. This acts as a protective barrier for my child's skin.

—Shilpa Amin-Shah, MD, a mom of a 6-year-old son and 5-year-old and 18-month-old daughters and an emergency medicine physician at Emergency Medical Associates, in St. Johns, FL

When your baby's behind is looking rosy, try soothing it with Triple Paste. It's a prescription-strength diaper rash cream that's gentle enough to use every day.

A two-ounce tube costs around $9, and you can buy it at Babies R Us, BuyBuyBaby, CVS, RiteAid, Target, Toy R Us, Walgreens, Walmart, and other fine retailers. For more information, visit TRIPLEPASTE.COM.

*The maker of Triple Paste is a paying partner of Momosa Publishing LLC. Regardless of whether we receive compensation from a vendor, we only recommend products or services that we have used personally and that we believe will be good for our readers.*

# Chapter 9

## Considering Sleep Training

We love a good oxymoron: Great Depression, jumbo shrimp, sleep training.

Here at the Mommy MD Guides, we aim to present options—not to force one person's opinion on every mom. Parenting is not a one-size-fits-all proposition. Every family is complex, with many moving parts. We encourage you to read about sleep training, talk with people you trust about it, and make the right decision for your baby, for yourself, and for your family. And know that what you decide today might not be the right decision tomorrow, next week, or next month. Exercise your parental prerogative to change your mind.

### JUSTIFICATION FOR A CELEBRATION

If you don't have to try sleep training, you will really feel like celebrating.

> **You cannot force sleep upon a baby. Creating a secure environment that allows sleep to overtake baby is the best way to create long-term healthy sleep attitudes. The frequent-waking stage will not last forever.**
>
> *—William Sears, MD,*
> **The Baby Book: Everything You Need to Know About Your Baby from Birth to Age Two**

## Avoiding Sleep Training

In one episode of *Jon and Kate Plus Eight*, Kate Gosselin described hearing her babies cries felt like "My brain is spinning around in my head." It's that primal urge to keep our babies happy that makes so many moms avoid sleep training like we avoid breastaurants.

While I have a lot of friends who sleep trained their children, my first child really drove the way I approached sleep with all three of my kids. Perhaps they "sleep trained" me instead.

> —*Sigrid Payne DaVeiga, MD, a mom of 10-year-old and 1-month-old sons and a 5-year-old daughter and a pediatric allergist with the Children's Hospital of Philadelphia, in Pennsylvania*

I was a resident in pediatrics when my third child was born. I was working 110 hours each week, breastfeeding, and feeling guilty. My hubby was the only other caregiver, and I sabotaged his sleep training because *I did not care*. When I got home, I wanted to see my baby, feel her, feed her, smell her.

> —*Hana R. Solomon, MD, a mom of four grown biological children, two grown "spiritually adopted" children, a grandmom of eight, a pediatrician, the president of BeWell Health, LLC, the inventor of Dr. Hana's Nasopure nose wash for children, and the author of* Clearing the Air One Nose at a Time: Caring for Your Personal Filter, *in Columbia, MO*

### ♥ Train Yourself for Better Sleep

Preparing for a better night of sleep often starts hours before you go to bed. To train yourself for better sleep, get some exposure to sunlight during the day, avoid stimulants such as caffeine and nicotine after 12 pm, don't take a nap after 3 pm, eat a light dinner, wind down with relaxing activities before bedtime, and take a hot bath, which will cause a drop in your body temperature afterward and help bring on sleepiness. Sleep tight!

My daughter hated being in her crib. I used many getting-the-baby-to-sleep crutches, such as nursing her to sleep and then sneaking her into bed.

Being a working mom, I spent so much time away from her. I felt

**BABY SLEEP PRO TIP:** Sleep Learning Methods

Sleep training is never one-size-fits-all. Here are some sleep training methods that work.

Once you make the decision to help your child sleep better—it usually hits you in the middle of the night after hundreds of wake-ups!—the next step is to commit to it by selecting a method that you think will work best for your child and your family. The good news is there are a variety of effective sleep training methods to choose from. The one that will work best depends on a variety of factors, including your child's temperament, your goals, your tolerance level, and the amount of involvement you would like to have in the process. In my experience, there is no one-size-fits-all sleep training method, because every child has a different temperament. Furthermore, every family has different routines and goals, so what works best for one family does not work for another.

The key to successful sleep learning is 100 percent consistency in implementing whatever method you choose. Don't give up if it doesn't seem to be working ater a day or two. Sometimes it takes a few weeks of consistency for your baby to learn the crucial skill of self-soothing.

Here are your options.

**Cry it out (CIO) aka "extinction":** Advocated by Marc Weissbluth, MD, extinction, more popularly known as "cry it out," is the method where you put your baby safely in his crib, close the door, and let him cry until he falls asleep. Although it takes the least parental involvement, it's not for the faint of heart, because the prolonged crying is hard for many families. The benefit is results happen fast, usually within days. For many parents, the

guilty about that, and I couldn't stand to hear her cry on top of it.

—*Lauren Hyman, MD, a mom of a 13-year-old daughter and an 11-year-old son and an ob-gyn at West Hills Hospital and Medical Center, in California*

benefits of having a well-rested baby and family outweigh the challenge of listening to the baby cry.

**Check and console aka "Ferberizing":** A slightly more gradual approach with more parental involvement was popularized by Richard Ferber, MD, in his book *Solve your Baby's Sleep Problems*. Also called "controlled crying," the method gradually increases the amount of time between checking on your baby (5 minutes, 10 minutes, 15 minutes, etc) until he falls asleep. Over the course of several nights, your child's crying will gradually diminish, and he will learn to fall asleep on his own. This method works for parents who can tolerate some crying, but prefer to reassure their child and themselves during the process.

**Fading aka the "chair method":** This method is even more gradual. It works especially well for parents who prefer not to let their babies cry alone. Instead, you sit on a chair progressively farther and farther away from the crib over the course of a couple of weeks until finally the chair is out of the room and then out of your baby's sight. Although you don't pick up your child in this method, you're in the same room to console him and offer reassurance.

**Pick up/put down:** This method, described by Tracy Hogg, sometimes called the Sleep Whisperer, requires intense parental participation. You pick up your baby every time she cries and then put her down as soon as she calms down. This is repeated over and over until she falls asleep. You usually have to repeat this method for several days and nights to succeed. But the method does work well for some parents, who feel it is the most "gentle" way to teach their babies to sleep.

**—Rebecca Kempton, MD**

I couldn't listen to my babies crying. A child's personality, and a parent's personality matters. When my babies were learning how to self soothe and fall asleep on their own, I would let them fuss for as long as I could stand. I sometimes put earplugs in and set a timer. I usually could only take it for five minutes.

Also, you know your babies' cries. If my baby was really in distress, I would go pick her up. If a baby is sick, teething, or having a growth spurt, she might cry more than normal. These aren't good times to try to get her to learn how to fall to sleep on her own.

—*Eva Mayer, MD, a mom of a 12-year-old daughter and an 11-year-old son, an associate professor of pediatrics at Temple University, and a pediatrician with St. Luke's Hospital Coopersburg Pediatrics, in Pennsylvania*

❧

I totally don't believe in letting a baby cry to get them used to sleeping "alone." It's the cruelest, most horrible method, the Ferber method.

A baby is a helpless being, dependent on everyone for everything. When babies cry, it's to say they need something. When babies cry and there's no response, the only psychological conclusion for them is a terrible sense of helplessness.

I always felt that comforting my child was reassuring him that the world is not a cruel and lonely place, and that there is nurturing and love for him. My son turned out to be a loving, secure human being with compassion toward others. I feel that being treated with compassion as a baby was instrumental in his becoming the way he is.

—*Judith Hellman, MD, a mom of an 18-year-old son, an associate clinical professor of dermatology at Mt. Sinai Hospital and a dermatologist in private practice, in New York City*

❧

I didn't expect my own children to "cry it out." But I did recognize that babies don't always have very consolidated sleep patterns. Many babies will wake up several times a night and fuss, whimper, or yell for a few moments before falling back asleep. Sometimes parents are reluctant to let a baby cry for even a minute before running in to pick up or soothe the baby. In my experience as a mother and as a physician, giving a baby a few moments to settle down and fall back asleep without interference is a sensible approach.

The "cry it out" method is controversial, although apparently scientific studies have shown that it is effective in helping many children who have already developed problematic sleep habits to achieve more restful sleep, and therefore improves their mood during the day.

—*Elizabeth Berger, MD, a mom of two grown children, a child psychiatrist, and the author of* Raising Kids with Character, *in New York City*

༄

With my older daughter, at some point when she was a toddler, I read the Ferber book. I tried to have her cry it out. I couldn't tolerate that approach. We both got too distressed, and we didn't make it past the first night. Mothers intuitively know that babies can't self-soothe. Our babies' cries distress us, and we want to jump in and help them stop. Infants are totally helpless and dependent. They rely on their parents for everything, including soothing.

To let a baby cry it out and figure out on its own how to calm down is counterintuitive. It's more natural for a mom to calm and comfort her baby.

A recent study confirmed mom's intuition to soothe her child is correct. The researchers found that soothing your baby creates a happier baby, which leads to a happier adult.

When you consistently work to meet your baby's needs, the infant learns that the world is a safe and nurturing place, and you help her to wire her brain in a positive and healthy way. On the other hand, if you leave a newborn without what she needs, such as water, food, or comfort, then she learns that the world is a scary, unpredictable place, and her brain wires up that way. These earliest experiences are crucial to developing a healthy brain and a positive attitude in the future.

—*Eva Ritvo, MD, a mom of two grown daughters, a psychiatrist, and a coauthor of* The Beauty Prescription *in Miami Beach, FL*

## Trying Sleep Training

For a myriad of reasons, many moms come to a place—sometimes one that feels like quiet desperation—of needing to sleep train. If you find yourself in this place, we hope you learn, as we did, that sometimes the end truly does justify the means.

⌒

My second baby was a much better sleeper than my first. I completely attribute the better sleeping to how we handled his first six months and when we did sleep training. We did it way too late with the first!

—*Heather Orman-Lubell, MD, a mom of 15- and 11-year-old sons and a pediatrician at St. Chris Care of Yardley Pediatrics, in Pennsylvania*

⌒

We didn't do the cry it out method until my twins were about 18 months of age. In hindsight, maybe we waited too long. Those first two years were exhausting.

—*Sonal R. Patel, MD, a mom of four-year-old twin daughters and a physician who specializes in pediatric/adult allergy and immunology with Adventist Health Physicians Network, in Los Angeles, CA*

⌒

I found the book *Solve Your Child's Sleep Problems*, by Richard Ferber, MD, was the best how-to on sleep training. Once a baby weighs 10 pounds, and is around six weeks old, he can be trained to sleep through the night.

—*Hana R. Solomon, MD*

⌒

When my first son was born, I was in medical school. I needed him to sleep so I could sleep. I used the Ferber method. I felt guilty about it, but I had to sleep. I was forced to be more aggressive about it than I wanted to be. It worked. My oldest slept through the night at a much younger age than my younger sons, whom I didn't sleep train. I didn't have as demanding a job then, so I could be more lenient with them.

—*Kristy Magee, MD, a mom of 15-, 12-, and 8-year-old sons and a family physician at North Seminole Family Practice and Sports Medicine, in Sanford, FL*

> **Remember, sleep training means starting to respect your baby's need to sleep when he is a newborn by anticipating when he will need to sleep (within one to two hours of wakefulness), learning to recognize drowsy signs, and developing a bedtime routine. Then your baby will not become overtired.**
>
> **—Marc Weissbluth,**
> **Healthy Sleep Habits, Happy Child**

When my baby was nine months old, in complete desperation, one night I let him cry it out. I was shocked that he slept! From that night on, he honed his self-soothing skills. Although we still cuddled at bedtime, he didn't need me anymore to fall asleep, and that made all the difference. He became a champion sleeper, and those sleepless nights eventually became a distant memory.

> —*Rebecca Kempton, MD, a mom of eight- and six-year-old sons and a three-year-old daughter and an infant and toddler sleep specialist, in Chicago, IL*

The most important thing to remember about any stage of parenting is it does get better. Also, babies don't die if they cry. As long as they are safe, fed, well, and clean, if they cry—even for an hour—they usually get tired and fall asleep.

However, it's important to remember that parents can get very frustrated, and babies *do* die from being shaken. If you're at your wit's end, put your baby in a safe place, such as her crib. Put on music. Close the door. Take a break. Check on the baby every 15 minutes or so.

Sometimes babies just need to cry, to decompress. We all would love to yell for an hour or two, but as we get older, we can't really do that.

> —*Sharon Boyce, MD, a mom of seven- and five-year-old sons and a family physician with Oaklawn Medical Group, in Albion and Bellevue, MI*

### Schedule a Phone Call During Sleep Training

Sleep training takes perseverance. One way to distract yourself from going back into your child's room—all the while getting some much-needed time to yourself—is to schedule a phone call with a friend or family member. Catching up with someone you're close to will help you feel more upbeat and help you keep to your sleep training schedule.

When a baby is six weeks old and weighs around 10 pounds, she should be able to sleep through the night. You are helping her to build good sleep hygiene and sleep discipline. A baby might sleep from 7:30 pm to 6 am or 9 pm to 7 am, for example.

After my babies had reached these milestones, when they woke up and cried, I would check to make sure they were okay. But I wouldn't feed them. They might cry for a bit. I would pat them on the back, give them a pacifier, and get out of the room. If a baby still cries despite these minor measures or even if the type of cry is different than usual, you have to assess the baby from head to toe, making sure you aren't missing anything.

Babies' sleep cycles are like ours. You wake up, toss around, and go back to sleep. Babies do the same; they're just louder! They cry for a million reasons, not just because they're hungry.

*—Aline T. Tanios Keyrouz, MD, a mom of 13- and 7-year-old and 9-month-old daughters and an 11-year-son and an assistant professor of pediatrics at St. Louis University, in Missouri*

After four years of raising a kid who thought Mommy was her sooth-ing "blankie" (I was frankly more like a slave conditioned to jump at her every whimper), my husband threatened to toss the evil baby monitor, if not his spouse, out the window. I finally read *Solve Your Child's Sleep Problems* by Dr. Richard Ferber. I realized I had failed my child by not allowing her to learn to self-soothe and fall sleep naturally.

All the sleep-promoting gadgets and gimmicks actually prevent a child from learning to self-soothe.

My husband and I embarked on Ferberizing our child, more than three years too late. After one brutal night when I literally put her to bed 73 times, she finally slept through the night—just in time for my twins to be born...

—*Susan Wilder, MD, a mom of a 22-year-old daughter and 17-year-old twins, a primary care physician, and the founder and CEO of LifeScape Premier, LLC, in Scottsdale, AZ*

We were a little late sleep training our baby. We had gotten into the habit of letting her sleep in a mechanical swing in our room when she was little. Then when we moved her to a crib in a separate room, we would go in and take her out of the crib every time she cried in the middle of the night. When she was around nine months old, we decided we had to train her to sleep through the night in the crib. We had one rough night when we put her in the crib and she cried the entire night. Needless to say, my husband and I didn't get much sleep that night!

But after that one night, our daughter started getting into a routine. When she would wake up crying, she would console herself and go back to sleep. The first time she slept through the night in her own crib was amazing!

—*Sonali Ruder, DO, a mom of a three-year-old daughter, an emergency medicine physician, and the author of* Natural Baby Food, *in Fort Lauderdale, FL*

Today my kids are terrific sleepers. I *truly* believe that it's because I've had them on sleep schedules—always!

I was one of those super-strict mommies who employed the "Babywise" approach—a very routine-based schedule. I know many moms find this method unimaginable, but during both my pregnancies and newborn periods, I was working, my husband was traveling, and my rheumatoid arthritis was in full swing. I've always been a schedule person, and more than ever at that time in my life I needed sanity—and sleep. A schedule was the only thing I could count on.

Nowadays, there's mounting evidence that our bodies work most efficiently when we're on a sleep schedule, even on the weekends. I have always believed that, but that notion was not always well accepted. Any mom who has had a cranky, emotional kid the day after a sleepover can see firsthand the effects of a disrupted sleep schedule!

—*Antoinette Cheney, DO, a mom of a 12-year-old son and an 11-year-old daughter, and a family physician with Rocky Vista University College of Osteopathic Medicine, in Parker, CO*

❧

Because I have a new baby and older kids, I have an interesting challenge. My older kids don't want to let the baby cry! When my baby would wake up and cry, they would go in to her room and pick her up. They didn't understand that she cries when she wants to sleep; you don't go in and pick her up!

One day, my baby cried, wanting attention, and she succeeded in getting it. All three of her siblings went to her, one at a time to her rescue, which is too cute to see that they care, but it doesn't help with sleep discipline.

When you have older kids, they need to follow your rules with the baby. I explained to my children that when the baby is in bed, no one touches her. She will fall asleep; leave her alone!

—*Aline T. Tanios Keyrouz, MD*

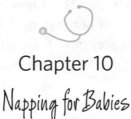

# Chapter 10

## Napping for Babies

In the United States, National Napping Day is March 14. We hope that in your house, every day is napping day.

In the United States, we sometimes call them "power naps." Other cultures have their own napping "nomikers":

- In Bengal, they take *bhat-ghum*, which means "rice sleep."
- Generally older people in Serbia and Slovenia call it a "house rule" where people know not to call or visit each other from 2 to 5 pm, when they're supposed to be resting.
- In northern India, a *sustana* means "taking a small nap."
- An afternoon sleep in China and Taiwan is called *wujaio*.
- Some German-speaking regions have a *Mittagspause*, during which shops close and children are urged to play indoors.
- And in Spain, of course, they call them *siestas*.

### JUSTIFICATION FOR A CELEBRATION

Any time you can get your baby to settle herself down for a nap, give yourself a big pat on the back.

> **I usually take one two-hour nap from one to four.**
>
> —*Yogi Berra*

## Napping at Home

In our hurry-scurry lives, it's not always possible for your baby to nap at home. But when all of the stars align and you're home at naptime, it's a great opportunity for your baby to get a good-quality nap in her own crib or bassinet—and for you to get some good-quality me time.

Here are some pointers to help ease your little one into naptime.

• Aim for consistent naptimes. Babies are creatures of habit!

• But be a little flexible. You want to hit that small window of opportunity where your baby is drowsy—when she has droopy blinky eyes and rubs her eyes and face—before she becomes overtired—when she's crying and grumpy.

• If your baby is still taking many 20-minute cat-naps throughout the day—not even time to catch up on *Grey's Anatomy!*—it's time to start consolidating those naps into fewer, longer naps. Try to keep your baby awake longer and slowly increase the amount of time between naps. You'll hopefully be rewarded with two-hour-long naps and better sleep at night too.

• Set the stage for sleep by making the room dark, quiet, and a comfortably cool temperature.

• Avoid rocking, walking, or nursing your baby to sleep at naptime, just like you do at bedtime.

• Follow the same safe sleeping steps as you would at night time: Put your baby to sleep on her back in her crib with no toys, bumpers, or blankets. Don't let your baby nap with other children or pets.

> **Let him sleep, for when he wakes,**
> **he will move mountains.**
>
> —*Napoleon*

At home, our babies always napped in their cribs.

> —*Shilpa Amin-Shah, MD, a mom of a 6-year-old son and 5-year-old and 18-month-old daughters and an emergency medicine physician at Emergency Medical Associates, in St. Johns, FL*

When our baby first came home, she napped in a Pack 'n Play in the living room close to the kitchen and the action.

> —*Katja Rowell, MD, a mom of a 10-year-old daughter, a family practice physician, and the author of* Helping Your Child with Extreme Picky Eating and Love Me, Feed Me *at TheFeedingDoctor.com, in St. Paul, MN*

My babies didn't go to day care. So when I went back to work, their nap locations and schedules didn't change. Their first babysitters were grandparents, and then we hired church members as nannies.

We simply told the sitters the napping schedules and locations we used, and they followed our instructions well.

> —*Sharon Boyce, MD, a mom of seven- and five-year-old sons and a family physician with Oaklawn Medical Group, in Albion and Bellevue, MI*

## Napping at Day Care

Few things are scarier than things being out of control. Certainly you did your homework and chose the safest day care you could find. Talk with the staff about their sleep safety procedures and check up on them as often as you feel comfortable.

According to the American Academy of Pediatrics, "About one in five Sudden Infant Death Syndrome (SIDS) deaths occurs while an infant is in the care of someone other than a parent. Many of these deaths occur when babies who are used to sleeping on their backs at home are then placed to sleep on their tummies by another caregiver … You can reduce your baby's risk of dying from SIDS by talking to those who care for your baby, including child care providers, babysitters, family, and friends, about placing your baby to sleep on his back during naps and at night."

Here are a few questions to ask your day care provider.
- Do all babies sleep in their own cribs?
- Are babies always placed to sleep on their backs, with nothing else in the crib?
- Is anything within reach of the babies' cribs, such as window blind cords, mobiles, or other cribs?
- Are babies directly supervised while they are asleep?

### Cherish Naptime

A mother's job is never done, which is why your baby's naptime should be something you hold dear to your heart.

If you're getting enough sleep at night and you no longer need to sleep when your baby is sleeping, now is your chance to use naptime for something you enjoy. Your baby may still be taking a couple of naps a day or might have graduated to a single nap that lasts two or three hours. Take some time for yourself during this time and have an uninterrupted phone conversation with a friend, watch your favorite TV show, use the time to meditate or practice yoga, write in a journal, or do anything that will help you relieve stress and feel good.

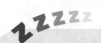

## BABY SLEEP PRO TIP
### Tips for the Two- to One-Nap Transition

**Time it right.** The average age for the transition is 15 to 18 months. Your child will shift to one afternoon nap starting between 12 and 1 pm, in sync with internal biological rhythms.

**Don't jump the gun.** If you do, you risk daytime melt-downs and night wakings as a result of the accumulated sleep debt.

**Recognize signs your child may be ready for one nap:**
• She consistently refuses one of her two naps over the course of several weeks.
• One of her two naps becomes much shorter—usually the afternoon nap.
• Your predictable nap schedule starts to go haywire, and sometimes she naps too late in the day.

**Be patient.** The transition can take a few weeks or more. It can be a challenge because your child is getting less sleep. Here are some tips.
• Cap the morning nap. Put your child down in the morning sometime between 9 and 10 am and cap the nap at 30 to 45 minutes. Decrease the length of the nap by 15 minutes over the course of a couple weeks. This catnap in the morning helps prevent your child from becoming too tired by the time of her afternoon nap.
• Put your child down for the second nap between 12 and 1 pm.
• Another strategy is to slowly move the morning nap later by 15 minute increments every few days until you reach a midday nap that begins between 12 and 1 pm and lasts for 1 to 2 hours.
• Compensate for less daytime sleep with an earlier bedtime temporarily, even 5:30 to 6 pm during the transition. Once your child has successfully shifted to one nap, you can go back to a later bedtime. A good rule of thumb is that bedtime should be about 4 to 4½ hours after the end of the nap, as long as it was a restorative 1- to 2-hour nap.

—*Rebecca Kempton, MD*

> **I count it as a certainty that in paradise, everyone naps.**
>
> —*Tom Hodgkinson*

My children started day care when they were 19 months old. They slept on a mat like the other children, but we also sent in blankets and pillows from home for them.

—*Shilpa Amin-Shah, MD*

## Napping on the Go

Moms are expert multi-taskers! So it might make sense to combine naptime with errand running. But consider this: How comfortably and well would you sleep in your car, sitting up on a relatively hard seat? Probably not too well.

On occasion, it's unavoidable, and your baby will fall asleep in the car—no doubt right as you're rounding that last corner for home. When that happens, simply carry your baby right in her carseat into your house. Set it safely on the floor—never on a table or couch. Leave your baby buckled in, and keep an eye on her, from where you are, hopefully able to do something fun and relaxing for yourself! Ah, naptime!

My children did nap in the car—a lot. I know this is very controversial, but we traveled a lot with our children. We often planned long car rides around their nap time because they slept very easily in the car.

We *never* put jackets on our babies in the car. Usually our nanny, my husband, or I sat in the back with the children.

—*Shilpa Amin-Shah, MD*

My babies didn't nap much in the car. But when their carseats were still rear-facing, I worried that they could have a problem, and I wouldn't know. I bought a mirror that attached to the car's seat. That way, I could look in the rearview mirror, and I could see their faces in the baby mirror.

> —Eva Mayer, MD, a mom of a 12-year-old daughter and an 11-year-old son, an associate professor of pediatrics at Temple University, and a pediatrician with St. Luke's Hospital Coopersburg Pediatrics, in Pennsylvania

## RALLIE'S TIP

*After the age of about eight months or so, my boys did much better napping on the go than they did when I put them down in their cribs for a nap, and that was fine with me! I'm not a highly structured person, so it was challenging for me to be at my house at nap time every single day.*

*My oldest son was a teenager when his brothers were born, and I didn't want his teenage years to be governed by his brothers' nap times. It was stressful enough for him to have two new babies in the house! So my younger boys learned to nap in their car seats on the way to karate lessons, and they napped in a double stroller at football practice. I liked knowing that I could count on my little boys to take a nap just about anywhere. It gave me the freedom to leave the house, and it made it possible for me to give my teenager the attention he needed at a critical time in his life.*

*Although my babies didn't always nap in their cribs, I tried to keep their naps at the same time every day, and I made sure they had a comfy, safe place to sleep, whether it was a car seat or a stroller. I also made sure I had everything they needed to get to sleep—a paci for one baby, and a lovey for the other.*

> From my observation, the older you get, the more you like the word cozy. That's why most of the elderly wear pants with elastic waistbands. If they wear pants at all. This may explain why grandparents are in love with buying grandkids pajamas and bathrobes.
>
> — *Holly Goldberg Sloan, film director and novelist*

# Chapter 11

## Focusing on Safe Sleeping

As your baby grows and develops, learning to roll over, sit up, crawl, and stand, keeping him safe becomes more of a challenge. Certainly, you chose the safest crib for your baby that you could find. But what about when you take the show "on the road"? When you're at your in-laws, a friend's, or a hotel, you might borrow a crib. Here are some important safety pointers to keep in mind.

- The crib slats must be no more than 2⅜ inch apart—you shouldn't be able to slide a soda can between them.
- The slats aren't broken or missing.
- Use a proper, fitted crib sheet—not an adult bed sheet.
- The crib mattress fits snugly, with no gaps between the mattress and the crib.
- The mattress is not soft, rather quite firm.
- There are no mobiles with strings hanging above the crib.
- No window blinds, strings, or curtains are within the baby's reach.

### JUSTIFICATION FOR A CELEBRATION

Sometime during your baby's first year, you will go into his room to check on him, and he will be standing in his crib, grinning from ear to ear. It will melt your heart!

## Keeping Toys and Blankets Out of the Crib

For 25 years, the American Academy of Pediatrics has urged parents to keep toys, blankets, pillows, and bumpers—anything soft other than your baby—out of the crib. It's also important to keep all child-carrying devices, recliners, and sleep positioners out of your baby's crib.

Just for fun (yes, we love our jobs!), we Googled images of "baby crib," expecting to find thousands of photos of baby cribs decorated with smooshy bumpers, soft blankets, fluffy pillows, and stuffed animals.

We were actually surprised to find page after page of images of cribs containing only fitted sheets! We love it when a plan comes together.

Certainly, we found some photos with a blanket artfully draped over the side of the crib, which we would like to think would have been removed by the imaginary photo mom before she put her imaginary photo baby into the crib.

Of course, you can *have* all of the baby blankets, stuffed animals, and pillows you want. Just keep them out of your baby's crib—for now.

### 🎯 Mommy MD Guides-Recommended Product
**Sweet Jojo Designs Chevron Gray and White Crib Bedding**

This crib set will work for a baby girl or boy. It offers a soft-brushed microfiber fabric in a modern chevron design.

A crib set includes a fitted sheet, crib skirt, blanket, diaper stacker, toy bag, decorative pillow, and two window valances for $265.99. For now, be sure to use the blanket and pillows as room decorations *outside* of your baby's crib.

You can buy it from the Sweet Jojo Designs website here:
**SWEETJOJODESIGNS.COM/CHEVRON-GY-WH-CRIB-BABY-BEDDING**

We only had a fitted sheet on the mattress and nothing else. No loose sheets, blankets, bumpers, or toys.

—*Sonali Ruder, DO, a mom of a three-year-old daughter, an emergency medicine physician, and the author of* Natural Baby Food, *in Fort Lauderdale, FL*

I didn't let our girls sleep with any toys, as per the American Academy of Pediatrics recommendations, until they were much older.

Now my daughters are seven and five years old, and they each have their favorite stuffed animal that they sleep with. I have to make sure I pack them on every vacation.

—*Jeannette Gonzalez Simon, DO, a mom of seven- and five-year-old daughters and a pediatric gastroenterologist, in Verona, NJ*

A key to being able to fall asleep is feeling safe and secure. When I put my babies to bed, I always tried to make sure they felt safe and secure and that their needs were met: They weren't hungry and didn't need a diaper change. Their environment was conducive to sleep: quiet and with the right temperature and level of light. And most important, there was nothing dangerous around: no toys in the crib or draperies within reach. This is crucial for baby—and Mom—to be able to sleep. Safety is of the utmost importance.

—*Eva Ritvo, MD, a mom of two grown daughters, a psychiatrist, and a coauthor of* The Beauty Prescription, *in Miami Beach, FL*

## Protect Your Sleep; Protect Your Health

Getting a good night's rest that's not disrupted by sleep apnea is very important. Sleep apnea puts you at risk for type 2 diabetes, high blood pressure, heart problems, and accidents. But you can prevent sleep apnea by losing excess weight, exercising regularly, avoiding medications that suppress your breathing, sleeping on your side, quitting smoking, and keeping your nasal passages clear.

**BABY SLEEP PRO TIP:** Ready to Roll

Once babies can roll over independently, it's okay to let them stay there and learn to fall asleep on their tummies per the American Association of Pediatrics.

—*Rebecca Kempton, MD*

I put my babies to sleep on their backs. However, once they could roll over by themselves from their backs to their tummies, I didn't wake them to flip them back! I didn't panic about it. I figured if they rolled over, they could roll back.

> —*Lauren Hyman, MD, a mom of a 13-year-old daughter and an 11-year-old son and an ob-gyn at West Hills Hospital and Medical Center, in California*

## Dressing the Baby for Sleep

Likely a step of your new sleep routine is dressing your little one in pajamas. Which pjs should you choose?

"The fabric of our lives" is a good option for baby's sleep. Cotton is breatheable and comfortable, making it a good choice for pajamas. The breathability factor is important for comfort as well as safety. It helps keep baby's body temp ideal during sleep.

As your baby gets older, you'll notice labels on pjs announcing if they are flame-retardant or if they must be worn tight fitting. That's because legally, any pajamas from size nine months through size 14 must be either flame-resistant or they must be tight fitting. Loose clothing more easily catches on fire.

Be sure your baby's sleepwear is free of any strangulation hazards, such as a hood or ties, or choking hazards like buttons. If you give your baby a pacifier to sleep with, make sure it doesn't have a cord.

Because you're not supposed to have blankets in the crib with the baby, his pajamas need to be warm. I bought baby footed pajamas. For winter, fleece pajamas are nice to keep the baby warm.

> —*Aline T. Tanios Keyrouz, MD, a mom of 13- and 7-year-old and 9-month-old daughters and an 11-year-son and an assistant professor of pediatrics at St. Louis University, in Missouri*

To keep my babies from overheating in summer, I dressed them in cotton summer pajamas and light cotton sleep sacks.

> —*Eva Mayer, MD, a mom of a 12-year-old daughter and an 11-year-old son, an associate professor of pediatrics at Temple University, and a pediatrician with St. Luke's Hospital Coopersburg Pediatrics, in Pennsylvania*

## Mommy MD Guides–Recommended Product
### Pajamagram

How much time do you spend buying, washing, folding, and dressing your little bundle of joy in his pajamas? We bet it's enough hours that you have earned a medal, a pony, or at least a new pair of pajamas!

Check out Pajamagram.com. This site promises you the "gift of relaxation." We love their "Leader of the Pack," "Mom is #1," "Fatigued," and "I Need Coffee" mom pjs. (Seriously, we *bought* their Leader of the Pack pjs!) All women's pajamas come with free gift packaging—a beautiful keepsake fabric gift bag that you could use to pack your adorable Momjamas on trips!

Pajamagram also sells matching "Mommy and Me," "His and Her," and "Matching Family" pajama sets—including pjs for Dad, Mom, kids, and even the family dog. Most of their women's pj sets cost $59.99. Visit **www.Pajamagram.com** for more information.

# Chapter 12

## Using Pacifiers and Sleep Toys

According to First Candle, an organization dedicated to Sudden Infant Death Syndrome (SIDS) prevention research and education, "Research shows that using a pacifier every time you place your baby down to sleep can greatly reduce the risk of SIDS. Doctors say that by using the following guidelines, pacifiers will not cause any problems for your baby.

"Some parents are hesitant to use a pacifier because of concerns about possible harmful effects, such as breastfeeding challenges, ear infections, and dental problems. Rest assured, research clearly shows that the potential benefits of pacifier use in reducing the risk of SIDS far outweigh any potential negative effects."

While it's perfectly okay to give your baby a pacifier right away, if you're concerned about breastfeeding, you could wait until your baby—and you!—really have the hang of nursing and offer a paci when your baby is around three weeks old.

It's important to note that you should not offer your baby a sleep toy—such as a stuffed animal or lovey—until your baby is able to roll over easily on her own. The logic is that before your baby can roll, she might get her face up against a soft toy or blanket and not be able to breathe. Once your baby can roll over, she'll be perfectly able to get away from stuffed Curious George or Barney in her sleep.

### JUSTIFICATION FOR A CELEBRATION
When your toddler gives up the pacifier is an excuse to celebrate!

## Choosing a Paci or Sleep Toy

Pacifiers have come a long way, baby! Many generations ago, pacifiers contained some pretty surprising substances, including lead, coral, and linen. Some were even dipped in whiskey or brandy!

In 1926, pacifiers were deemed to be unsanitary and banned in France. (The French are not big fans of the "five-second rule" apparently.) Today though, French moms probably have just as many pacifier options as moms elsewhere.

Here are some things to consider when choosing a pacifier.

- Buy a pacifier free of latex, to which babies can develop an allergy.
- Look for pacifiers free of BPA, PVC, and phthalates.
- Choose a pacifier designed for your baby's age.
- Make sure the pacifier has a vented shield at least 1½ inches wide to prevent choking.
- Don't buy a pacifier with any beads or decorations that could fall off and become choking hazards.

When choosing a sleep toy—which is safe to introduce after your baby can roll over—look for a stuffed animal or lovey that's around the same size as your baby's head. Avoid any buttons or decorations. Consider washability; it's best if you can machine wash the lovely, which is certain to come into contact with all bodily fluids, dirt, food, and anything else near your baby.

Our baby used the pacifier that they gave us at the hospital. I don't think hospitals give them out as regularly these days, though!

—*Katja Rowell, MD, a mom of a 10-year-old daughter, a family practice physician, and the author of* Helping Your Child with Extreme Picky Eating and Love Me, Feed Me *at TheFeedingDoctor.com, in St. Paul, MN*

Only one of our four babies used a pacifier. I was sick after she was born, and I think her dad introduced it to her to comfort her. We took it away when she was about three years old, and she got over it almost immediately. Like so many parenting things, I found it ended up being a bigger deal to us in our minds than to the children in reality.

> —*Rebecca Jeanmonod, MD, a mom of 12- and 8-year-old daughters and 11- and 8-year-old sons and a professor of emergency medicine and the associate residency program director for the emergency medicine residency at St. Luke's University Health Network, in Bethlehem, PA*

We used a pacifier. My daughter only liked the one that was given to us at the hospital. We bought two dozen of them! We put one in every car and space where our daughter would be. My husband used to call them "e-pacis"—as in E for emergency. He had one in his daddy diaper bag and his work car console.

> —*Lisa M. Campanella-Coppo, MD, a mom of a six-year-old daughter and an emergency department physician at Summit Medical Group, in Livingston, NJ*

Both of my babies used pacifiers. I've heard a lot of people worry that pacifiers impact nursing. I have not seen that to be the case. If after a baby nurses with good latch, non-nutritive sucking helps a baby to self-soothe.

Once I was checking on a newborn at the hospital. She was crying, and despite the nurses' best efforts, she wouldn't settle down. The nurses said, "She cries like this after every feeding."

I gave the baby a pacifier, and she was fine! She fell asleep, and she took a good nap. In two hours, she nursed again beautifully. Pacifiers are helpful for exhausted moms whose babies are using their nipples as a pacifier, latching and falling right asleep instead of drinking.

> —*Eva Mayer, MD, a mom of a 12-year-old daughter and an 11-year-old son, an associate professor of pediatrics at Temple University, and a pediatrician with St. Luke's Hospital Coopersburg Pediatrics, in Pennsylvania*

## Mommy MD Guides-Recommended Product
### Difrax Pacifiers

I tested the 18 month+ dental pacifiers by Difrax, and I recommend them to other parents. When my daughter was 19 months old, she still liked to use a pacifier. She enjoyed the Difrax pacifier, sometimes sucking on it and sometimes chewing on it.

I like it because it's designed to stimulate the development of her palate, tongue, and jaw muscles. I also like the unique butterfly shape that keeps her nose clear so that she can breathe properly. The colors and designs are also very bright and cheerful, which are a plus!

— Sonali Ruder, DO, a mom of a three-year-old daughter, an emergency medicine physician, and the author of *Natural Baby Food*, in Fort Lauderdale, FL

The Difrax pacifiers 6 months+ are really cute with fun colors and prints. The shape of the pacifier nipples is supposed to be friendly to baby's mouth development and easy to breathe with.

—Julie Graves, MD, PhD a mom of one daughter and a family medicine and public health physician

Difrax pacifiers have a unique, butterfly-shaped shield, and they come in trendy print designs and cheerful colors. The butterfly shape creates a natural recess, leaving the baby's nose unobstructed. This automatically helps your baby learn to breathe properly through her nose. The openings on either side of the shield allow air to flow between the shield and your baby's delicate skin, preventing irritation. Difrax pacifiers are available in five sizes, to keep pace with your baby's growth, from newborn to 18 months and over. The larger pacifiers come with larger shields too. The nipple is larger and stronger as well, to match your child's stronger jaws. Difrax pacifiers retail for $5.99 online at DIFRAX-USA.com. For more information visit us-en.DIFRAX.com.

My first baby was a pacifier kid. He needed his pacifier to soothe him. Nothing else would do for him, until he latched on to a small stuffed snowman when he was around six months old. Fifteen years later, that stuffed snowman is still on his bed.

My second baby was a blankie boy. He loved a small receiving blanket that he started using when he was around six months old. Eleven years later, it's in tatters, but it's still on his bed.

—*Heather Orman-Lubell, MD, a mom of 15- and 11-year-old sons and a pediatrician at St. Chris Care at Yardley Pediatrics, in Pennsylvania*

☙

Transitional objects, such as blankies or stuffed animals, help children learn to soothe themselves as they transition away from needing the parent to soothe them. My oldest carried around a blanket and rubbed the corner to calm down.

—*Eva Ritvo, MD, a mom of two grown daughters, a psychiatrist, and a coauthor of* The Beauty Prescription, *in Miami Beach, FL*

☙

When my kids were babies, they each had a small, soft thin blanket for transitional objects. I know some kids love those little blankets with stuffed animal heads on them. One mom in my practice bought five of them and passed them off to her baby as the same one!

It's safe to have these small thin blankets in the crib after a baby is four to six months old. The baby can roll over on her own by then.

—*Eva Mayer, MD*

☙

We didn't use pacifiers during the night with our babies. We wanted to teach our babies to pacify on their own with their hand or finger. This way, the pacifier couldn't get lost and require one of us to come in and find it for her. During the day and for naps, we gave our babies pacifiers if needed.

—*Marcela Dominguez, MD, a mom of a 13-year-old daughter and an 11-year-old son who has a private family medicine and wellness practice in Southern California, whose concierge medicine services are provided by Signature MD*

## Buying Multiples

This is the stuff mom nightmares are made of! You find the perfect lovey. Your baby loves the lovey. *You* love the lovey. The lovey goes along on an errand, never to be seen again. Your baby never sleeps again. *You* never sleep again.

Save yourself from this painful mom rite of passage and buy many multiples!

~

We had *lots* of pacifiers! They were everywhere!
—*Susan Besser, MD, a mom of six grown children, a grandmom of five, and a family physician at River Family Physicians, in Easton, MD*

~

I know that some dentists frown on pacifiers, but we felt that as a family, we needed our daughter to be able to sooth herself and sleep. Our family history is such that we all needed braces anyway, so we figured worrying about the paci was a moot point.
—*Lisa m. Camanella-Coppo, MD*

~

As our daughter got older, she slept with a few small plush toys. One was a penguin, and she liked to suck on the beak; another was a caterpillar that she sucked on. Then she chose one little guy as her favorite. We immediately bought two more of the same toy! I had seen my cousins spending hours many nights searching for a certain bedtime lovey for a toddler who wouldn't sleep without it. I didn't want to have to do that! I was so glad we had the spares.
—*Katja Rowell, MD*

> **When I go away to do a movie, I bring the blanket I've had since I was a little girl. It helps me sleep.**
>
> **—*Kirsten Dunst, actress***

## Giving Up the Paci

If your baby uses a pacifier, you're probably wondering when to have her give it up. This is one of those MomEnts that seem so critical at the time but will pale in hindsight. Your child will not take her pacifier to college. We promise.

You actually have several terrific windows of opportunity to give up the pacifier. They include the following.

- When your baby is six months old. This balances the time when SIDS risk drops but ear infection risk increases.
- When your child is two years old. That's when most toddlers start to give a pacifier up voluntarily.

My first baby used a pacifier. We took it away from him when he was two years old. We were lucky enough that when the dentist told him to give it up, he did!.

—*Heather Orman-Lubell, MD, a mom of 15- and 11-year-old sons and a pediatrician at St. Chris Care at Yardley Pediatrics, in Pennsylvania*

When our daughter was three years old, we decided the sleep paci had to go. It was beginning to displace her teeth. She only used it for sleep at that time. We had a "pacifier fairy" who came and took the pacis for children who needed them. It was surprisingly easy for us, for whatever reason! Within a few months, her teeth were fine.

—*Katja Rowell, MD*

My children both used pacifiers until they were around four months old. I knew at that point they didn't need the paci anymore. They were happy to replace it with a lovey. It wasn't hard to have them give it up at that point. When I took away the paci, my son simply started sucking his thumb instead.

The pacifier needs to be gone by the time a child is two years old, or else it starts affecting her teeth and can contribute to ear infections.

—*Eva Mayer, MD*

## Mommy MD Guides–Recommended Product
### Aden + Anais Blankets

We used the Aden + Anais blankets. I love them. They get softer every time you wash them. They are my go-to baby shower gift—every time.

My 18-month-old uses an Aden + Anais blanket as her comfort blanket now. Three kids and six years later, it's still super soft!
> —Shilpa Amin-Shah, MD, a mom of a
> 6-year-old son and 5-year-old and 18-month-old
> daughters and an emergency medicine physician
> at Emergency Medical Associates, in St. Johns, Florida

Aden + Anais classic blankets are made from 100 percent cotton muslin, a gentle and breathable fabric, while their silky soft muslin blankets are rayon made from bamboo. You can also choose blankets made from organic cotton.

A classic swaddle blanket costs $14, a set of two 16-inch x 16-inch security blankets (so your little one doesn't go without when the first blanket needs to be washed) costs $19.95, and the 47-inch x 47-inch dream blanket costs $54.95.

The blankets can be purchased from the Aden + Anais website at **ADENANDANAIS.COM.**

# Chapter 13
## Tweaking the Routine

Different ages call for different stages. In the United States, only 15 percent of babies are in out-of-the-home day care, but that number increases to 26 percent of one- and two-year-olds and 30 percent of three- and four-year-olds. When you or your partner go back to work and/or when your baby starts day care, it's likely to create a Teutonic shift in your routine.

Some people love and embrace change. Others try to avoid it like the plague. When all else fails, try to remember this: Sometimes change can be good, and sometimes different is better.

## JUSTIFICATION FOR A CELEBRATION
It's a fact of life: Just when your plan comes together, it falls apart. When you handle this bump in the road with grace, you deserve a treat.

> **The secret to your future is hidden in your daily routine. You have to be self-disciplined to spend your time wisely.**
>
> —*Michelle Moore*

## Adjusting the Routine

The one constant in parenting is change. Just when you adjust to a phase, it's replaced by an equally maddening one. Parenting isn't so much a dance as a sport, where you're constantly adjusting and flexing and learning and changing.

By the time your baby is a few months old, he's probably settled into a routine. Shortly thereafter, something will happen so the routine you've grown to love no longer works. Maybe you have gone back to work, or your baby has started day care. Some change in your life has necessitated a change in routine.

When you can, anticipate the change that's coming and adjust your baby's routine in small—say 10 minute—increments.

When my baby was about 15 months old, we changed our bedtime routine. It now consisted of tooth brushing, face washing and bathing, and then story time.

—*Michelle Davis-Dash, MD, a mom of a five-year-old son and a pediatrician, in Baltimore, MD*

Our daughter always slept less than the "recommended" amount of time—usually about one to two hours less. I worried at first that she wasn't getting enough sleep, but she slept soundly, woke on her own, and was happy and active upon waking. Overall her mood was really good when she was awake, and she didn't fall asleep randomly while we were out and about or while she was eating meals.

 **Save a Few Tasks for the Kids' Bedtime**

After the kids are quiet in their beds, taking the time to do a little housecleaning—such as washing the last of the dishes, straightening up, sweeping the floor, and putting out the trash—can make a busy next morning go more smoothly. It's also a great time to write out your schedule or put together a checklist for the next day.

Try to remember that "recommended" or "typical" ranges for sleep (or how much babies eat for that matter) are just that—*ranges*. Some children do well with less; others need more. Responding to your child's needs and what she communicates with her behaviors is most important. If your baby is having trouble with behavior or seems antsy, maybe trying an earlier bedtime or more of a regular routine is worth a try.

—*Katja Rowell, MD, a mom of a 10-year-old daughter, a family practice physician, and the author of* Helping Your Child with Extreme Picky Eating and Love Me, Feed Me *at TheFeedingDoctor.com, in St. Paul, MN*

## Baby Starting Day Care

You might be surprised to know that some babies actually sleep better at day care than they do at home! These babies might thrive on the stimulation and structure of day care. But on the other hand, some babies sleep better at home. These little ones might need more quiet and simply long to sleep in their own cribs.

Either way, when your baby starts to go to day care, you're going to notice some shift in her sleep at home—for worse or hopefully for better. The reality is, you probably can't impact the day care's schedule or facilities much. So it might be easier and more effective if you tweak your home routine to match the day care's. For example, you can ask for their nap schedule and ask if they listen to CDs or white noise.

‿◦‿

My children started nursery school for a couple of hours each day once they were two years old. Fortunately, it had no impact on their sleep.

—*Elizabeth Berger, MD, a mom of two grown children, a child psychiatrist, and the author of* Raising Kids with Character, *in New York City*

When my daughter started day care, her sleep routine changed. Instead of her being able to wake up naturally, I had to wake her to get her ready for day care. That caused a lot of cranky mornings until she adjusted.

Also I tended to keep my daughter up later in the evening after I got home from work so I could have more time with her. This resulted in a longer naptime during the day.

—*Kathryn Boling, MD, a mom of two grown daughters, a grandmom of two, and a family medicine physician with Mercy Medical Center, in Baltimore, MD*

When my babies started day care, we were careful not to change their routine at home. We were very strict about establishing a bedtime routine and sticking to it.

—*Shilpa Amin-Shah, MD, a mom of a 6-year-old son and 5-year-old and 18-month-old daughters and an emergency medicine physician at Emergency Medical Associates, in St. Johns, FL*

### Keeping a Sleep Journal or Log

When you're the one who can't seem to sleep through the night, a sleep journal could help you puzzle out what's keeping you up. Looking at your daily and nightly routine, such as when you exercise and when you turn off electronic devices, could help you understand what's disrupting your sleep patterns. A sleep journal is also handy to have if you need to see a doctor about insomnia.

You can find a free printable sleep diary from the National Sleep Foundation here: **SLEEPFOUNDATION.ORG/SLEEP-DIARY/ SLEEPDIARYV6.PDF**. It helps you track what time you went to bed and woke up, what disturbed your sleep, and things that could have affected your sleep, such as caffeine, exercise, and medications.

> **Fatigue is the best pillow.**
> *—Benjamin Franklin*

When my son was 18 months old, he started day care. I found out the details about the day care's schedule. Several months before he started there, I started to transition him to a schedule just like his school so he could get used to it.

> —*Larissa Guerrero, MD, a mom of a three-year-old son and family practice physician with Healthrow Ob/Gyn, in Orlando, FL*

## Keeping the Baby Busy During the Day to Sleep at Night

Who doesn't have the memory of being a child and having an endless summer day, building sand castles on the beach, playing in the surf, catching ice cream drips off a cone with your tongue, and collapsing into bed at night—where you had the deepest sleep of your life!

Therein lies the simple strategy of keeping your baby busy and active in the hopes he sleeps better at night!

I notice that if we play outside a lot during the day, my son sleeps better. I think it's because he's tired.

> —*Larissa Guerrero, MD*

Our boys definitely needed tiring out sometimes in order to be able to sleep. Sometimes we would keep them up for some special time with extra reading, play wrestling, or singing songs, just so they could be on the same schedule as we were, but that was when they were much older. In the end, when they were sleepy, they would fall asleep, and no one could stop them!

> —*Leena S. Dev, MD, a mom of teenage boys and a general pediatrician, in Maryland*

> **A well-spent day brings happy sleep.**
> *—Leonardo da Vinci*

I tried to keep my baby entertained and busy during the day to tire her out so she would sleep better at naps and at night. This was also important for her development: speech, motor, and behavioral. Because infants reach milestones at different times, I focus on interacting with them with age-appropriate activities, such as playing with blocks and reading books.

*—Aline T. Tanios Keyrouz, MD, a mom of 13- and 7-year-old and 9-month-old daughters and an 11-year-son and an assistant professor of pediatrics at St. Louis University, in Missouri*

We all know that exercise helps both children and adults get a better night's sleep. I found that when my son has an active day playing sports or swimming, he sleeps better at night.

On the flip side, if my son doesn't have a lot of activity during the day, it can be "crazy town" in the evening and at night.

*—Lauren Hyman, MD, a mom of a 13-year-old daughter and an 11-year-old son and an ob-gyn at West Hills Hospital and Medical Center, in California*

It didn't cross my mind to try to tire my babies out to help them to sleep better at night.

*—Elizabeth Berger, MD*

We tried to keep our babies busy to tire them out. But we felt it had the opposite result. It seemed that if our kids hit the "too tired" threshold, it was tougher to get them to sleep. I found the best strategy was just to keep to a regular nap/sleep schedule as best as possible.

*—Jennifer Bacani McKenney, MD, a mom a five-year-old daughter and a three-year-old son and a family physician, in Fredonia, KS*

# Chapter 14

## Changing and Growing

Like grass in springtime, you can practically see babies grow. In your baby's first year, the chances are good she'll triple her birth weight. She might grow eight inches taller.

In just one year, your baby's vocabulary will probably grow from zero words to saying a few words and understanding more than 100. She'll advance from hardly being able to control her head, arms, and legs to sitting, crawling, walking, and soon running!

Imagine if you were able to change and grow that much in a single year! You could change the world!

As your baby changes and grows, it only makes sense that her sleep will be affected. Some changes might actually help her sleep better (hurray!), while others will undoubtedly make her sleep worse. Similar to life in general, parenting is like a box of chocolates: Some phases turn out to be the gooey nougat, while others are the Bing cherries.

### JUSTIFICATION FOR A CELEBRATION

When you see that first tiny tooth peeking through the gums, it's time to celebrate and to start saving up for the Tooth Fairy fees!

> **Cleaning your house while your kids are still growing up is like shoveling the walk before it stops snowing.**
>
> *—Phyllis Diller*

## Introducing Solids and Sleep

Conventional wisdom says that babies sleep better after they start eating solid food. Many parents, desperate for sleep, start solids early in the hopes that this is true.

Several studies, however, have proved this to be a myth. These studies found that babies given solids at an earlier age don't sleep better than babies who weren't given solids.

While some babies do sleep better after starting solids, other babies sleep worse. They regress because of the change in their routines or because the new foods upset their bellies. A baby who had been sleeping through the night might suddenly be up a few times.

The American Academy of Pediatrics recommends starting solids when your baby is six months old. Earlier, it's best to nurse exclusively. Later, your baby might be more reluctant to try new foods. (Ha, wait until she's a toddler!)

Per the American Academy of Pediatrics, babies exclusive breastfed should not be offered solids until six months of age to get the full benefits of nursing. Rules are great, but not every family fits every rule. You have to be flexible.

When my kids were babies, I introduced solids when they were four months old. I went by my own children's developmental cues for readiness. They could sit in a high chair, started to wake up at night hungry when before they slept through the night, doubled their birthweight, looked and reached for food, and had good abdominal muscle control. I found that solids helped them to sleep better.

—*Eva Mayer, MD, a mom of a 12-year-old daughter and an 11-year-old son, an associate professor of pediatrics at Temple University, and a pediatrician with St. Luke's Hospital Coopersburg Pediatrics, in Pennsylvania*

> **One cannot think well, love well, sleep well, if one has not dined well.**
>
> —*Virginia Woolf, writer*

**Stay in the Dark**
Darkness triggers your body's release of melatonin, the hormone that helps you feel sleepy and can lead to a restful night of sleep.

If anything, starting solid foods helped my daughter sleep longer at night. She used to wake up every night at 2 am and again around 5 or 6 am. After she was eating solids, we gradually phased out the 2 am feeding, which meant more sleep for us!

—*Sonali Ruder, DO, a mom of a three-year-old daughter, an emergency medicine physician, and the author of* Natural Baby Food, *in Fort Lauderdale, FL*

For most of our children, introducing solid foods made them sleep longer. I think that's probably because the body has to work harder to digest solid foods, so babies stay fuller longer.

My second baby was a preemie, and he didn't adjust very well to solids. He resisted eating, worked himself up until he became upset, and had a harder time sleeping. I just had to wait until he was ready for solid foods. He ended up being exclusively breastfed for longer than six months, and we had to introduce foods very slowly with him.

—*Rebecca Jeanmonod, MD, a mom of 12- and 8-year-old daughters and 11- and 8-year-old sons and a professor of emergency medicine and the associate residency program director for the emergency medicine residency at St. Luke's University Health Network, in Bethlehem, PA*

## RALLIE'S TIP

*I breastfed my babies, and with each one, I tried to hold off introducing solid foods until they were at least four months old. When they were three months old, I was counting the days! All of my babies slept better once they started cereal. But I knew that if I gave them solids before they were old enough to handle them, they'd sleep worse, not better. So I waited, and counted the days!*

I gave my 15-month-old daughter several of the Ella's Kitchen Organic Baby Meal pouches. Before that, I had been making all of my daughter's baby food myself because I like using healthy ingredients and knowing what is in the food I give her.

When I read about Ella's Kitchen, I was impressed by the quality of the ingredients and the unique flavor combinations. I love the fact that Ella's Kitchen uses all-natural, USDA-certified organic ingredients. To my delight, my daughter loved all of the Ella's Kitchen Baby food pouches that we tried. I usually have a hard time getting my daughter to eat vegetables, but she loved the Pears Peas + Broccoli pouch!

I highly recommend Ella's Kitchen Organic 1, 2, and 3 Stage Baby Food pouches to other parents. With Ella's Kitchen, you know that you're getting only the highest quality ingredients. The flavor and ingredient combinations are unique, and my baby really enjoys them. Feeding your baby these pouches is a great way to make sure your baby gets a wide variety of important nutrients and flavors.

—Sonali Ruder, DO, a mom of a three-year-old daughter, an emergency medicine physician, and the author of *Natural Baby Food*, in Fort Lauderdale, FL

The Ella's Kitchen Organic mission is to develop healthy eating habits that last a lifetime by offering a range of healthy, handy and fun products. Their products are unsweetened and unsalted, do not use genetically modified ingredients, are made with fruit and veg purees not concentrates, contain no artificial colors, flavors or preservatives, and are made with unique ingredients and variety of flavors.

You can buy Ella's Kitchen Organic 1, 2, and 3 Baby Food pouches at stores such as Target, Whole Foods Market, and select Walmarts for around $1 to $3. Visit **WWW.ELLASKITCHEN.COM** for more information.

## Teething and Sleep

It's not difficult to imagine why teething would make it hard for your baby to sleep. Teething hurts! Just like you can't sleep if you have a toothache, your baby's sleep is affected by teething pain.

This is a case where you can treat the symptom (teething pain) to improve the result (poor sleep). Tried and true remedies include cool teething rings, massaging your baby's gums, over-the-counter pain medicine, and some brandy—for *you*, not your baby.

This is a great time for extra love, hugs, and kisses. Who are we kidding? It's *always* a great time for extra love, hugs, and kisses!

❧

When my babies started teething at about six or seven months old, they would sometimes wake if they were fussy, but teething medicine would help with this. For us, Camilia Drops and Hyland's Baby Teething Tablets seemed to be helpful.

—*Manpreet K. Gill, MD, a mom of a five-year-old daughter and a three-year-old son and a family practice physician with North Seminole Family Practice, in Sanford, FL*

❧

When my babies were teething, it completely threw off their sleeping and eating cycles. My oldest got a new tooth every month. When she was completely inconsolable, I gave her some Tylenol (acetaminophen). Otherwise, I let her suck on cold teething toys. Something that really worked was frozen fruit, put it in a mesh teething basket and given to her to suck on. This worked the best. Fair warning, it's very messy, but if I had a happy baby, I didn't mind.

—*Jeannette Gonzalez Simon, DO, a mom of seven- and five-year-old daughters and a pediatric gastroenterologist, in Verona, NJ*

❧

One of the biggest challenges of parenting is just when you've solved a problem, like getting your baby to sleep, something new comes along, like teething, and you have a bad night. It's easy to feel betrayed and think, *I thought we were past this!*

Try not to get discouraged. It's easy to feel overwhelmed and frustrated because you remember how exhausted you were the last time your baby didn't sleep. Remember that this is a minor setback, not a major derailment.

When my babies were teething and it affected their sleep, I gave them a dose of Tylenol (acetaminophen). It usually helped.

—*Deborah Gilboa, MD, a mom of 14-, 12-, 10-, and 8-year-old sons, a family physician with Squirrel Hill Health Center, in Pittsburgh, PA, and a parenting speaker whose advice is found at AskDoctorG.com*

I can't remember exactly when it started, but I know that we didn't sleep consistently from the time that my daughter was three months old until she was well past two years old.

Part of the problem was colic, but it was also teething. I used to give my daughter Tylenol (acetaminophen), and when she was old enough, I gave her Motrin (ibuprofen).

I remember feeling sorry for moms who weren't doctors because my daughter would pull her ears and scream when she was teething.

### Have Fun, Get Your Heart Rate Up

Much research has been done proving that exercise helps improve sleep. As your baby gets older, you may find you have more time to get out of the house for an hour or more for a workout. In one study published in 2012, researchers studied people who had trouble sleeping and found that those who started an exercise program reported better sleep quality.

Do something fun that feels more like a release rather than a workout. Try one of the latest trends in fitness, such as a Bollywood dance class, belly dancing, a barre class that uses ballet techniques, or a pound class that involves simulated drumming. If you don't have trendy classes in your area, go with a classic that you'll enjoy, such as Zumba, kickboxing, or spinning.

## Mommy MD Guides-Recommended Product
### FeverAll Acetaminophen Suppositories

If a baby refuses or is unable to take liquid acetaminophen for fever or pain, FeverAll is a great choice. I recommend FeverAll Acetaminophen Suppositories when babies are vomiting and not able to tolerate taking acetaminophen by mouth because they're given rectally, rather than orally.

> —Eva Mayer, MD, a mom of a 12-year-old daughter and an 11-year-old son, an associate professor of pediatrics at Temple University, and a pediatrician with St. Luke's Hospital Coopersburg Pediatrics, in Pennsylvania

Suppositories are a great option for when oral acetaminophen won't go or stay down. Parents will know their child received the exact dosage of acetaminophen required for their age every time.

FeverAll Acetaminophen Suppositories are available in infants, childrens, and junior strength at drugstores. For children up to age three, use the infants' strength of 80 milligrams, unless otherwise instructed by your doctor. FeverAll Infants' Strength is the only acetaminophen suppository approved for infants as young as six months.

FeverAll costs approximately $7 for a pack of six. For more information on FeverAll Acetaminophen Suppositories, visit **FEVERALL.COM**.

*The maker of FeverAll Acetaminophen Suppositories is a paying partner of Momosa Publishing LLC. Regardless of whether we receive compensation from a vendor, we only recommend products or services that we have used personally and that we believe will be good for our readers.*

If I hadn't been able to look in her ears to make sure she didn't have an ear infection, we would have been at the pediatrician's office almost weekly.

> —*Lisa M. Campanella-Coppo, MD, a mom of a six-year-old daughter and an emergency department physician at Summit Medical Group, in Livingston, NJ*

When my babies were teething, I wet washcloths and placed them in the freezer for a few minutes. Then I gave them to my babies to suck on. I also rubbed their gums. I sometimes gave them pieces of frozen banana to chew on.

I didn't give my babies any medicine for teething. Life is hard with plenty of painful conditions, such as menses and bruised knees. We must learn to tolerate life, not medicate.

I expected a bit of crabbiness when my babies were teething. But it didn't interfere with their sleep. Teething is often blamed for many infant issues—runny nose, fever, fussiness, and diarrhea. Teething is rarely or never the culprit of serious issues.

—*Hana R. Solomon, MD, a mom of four grown biological children, two grown "spiritually adopted" children, a grandmom of eight, a pediatrician, the president of BeWell Health, LLC, the inventor of Dr. Hana's Nasopure nose wash for children, and the author of* Clearing the Air One Nose at a Time: Caring for Your Personal Filter, *in Columbia, MO*

# Chapter 15

## Calming Colic

Colic. The word strikes fear in the hearts of moms-to-be. About 40 percent of babies develop colic. If yours is one of them, we feel for you. Ours did too.

The cause of colic is unknown. Perhaps that's because it can be caused by several different things. Some babies might cry inconsolably because they are super sensitive. Any deviation from status quo might make them uncomfortable. So if your baby is too hot, too cold, too wet, too dry, too anything-other-than-normal, she might cry. It's like Goldilocks on steroids.

Other babies might cry because their bellies hurt. In this case, if you're breastfeeding, colic might be a sign of sensitivity to a food that you're eating. Or maybe your baby is sensitive to a milk protein in her formula. Talk with your doctor or your baby's pediatrician about ways that tweaking your diet or changing your baby's formula might help. In any event, may the crying soon stop.

### JUSTIFICATION FOR A CELEBRATION

The day when your colicky baby suddenly isn't, you'll feel like the rain has finally stopped, the sun has come out, and all of the birds are singing with joy.

> **Crying is cleansing. There's a reason for tears —happiness or sadness.**
>
> *—Dionne Warwick*

## Recognizing Colic

Colic can be called the "condition of threes" because babies who have it often cry more than three hours a day, three days a week for three weeks or longer. Moms with babies who have colic often cry a whole lot more than that.

Probably the only good thing we can say about colic is it *will* end. For the rest of your life, when you tell people your baby had colic you will be rewarded with sympathetic looks from other moms.

My oldest child had colic. I was a first-time, inexperienced mom. Her crying was very disturbing. I knew it was colic because her crying spells came in clusters at night. If she was being carried, she was occasionally consolable.

She would have a crying spell for a few hours, which is always overwhelming to any mom. You feel helpless and your child is uncomfortable and upset. Fortunately, not all kids develop colic, and if they do, it usually lasts for one to two months.

—*Aline T. Tanios Keyrouz, MD, a mom of 13- and 7-year-old and 9-month-old daughters and an 11-year-son and an assistant professor of pediatrics at St. Louis University in Missouri*

When my daughter was about a month old, she started having nightly episodes of inconsolable crying. She cried every night from around 6 pm to 10 pm. I recognized that it was colic because it was so consistent.

It's very difficult and frustrating when your baby cries like that, night after night. I remember one night, holding her above my head with straight arms. I just looked at her and asked, "What on earth do you want?"

—*Eva Mayer, MD, a mom of a 12-year-old daughter and an 11-year-old son, an associate professor of pediatrics at Temple University, and a pediatrician with St. Luke's Hospital Coopersburg Pediatrics, in Pennsylvania*

> **There was never a child so lovely,**
> **but his mother was glad to get him to sleep.**
>
> —*Ralph Waldo Emerson,*
> *American essayist and lecturer*

My older daughter had colic. She started crying at around two weeks of age and cried every night for hours until we identified the problem and corrected it. Once my daughter got past her colic, she was a good sleeper.

> —*Eva Ritvo, MD, a mom of two grown daughters, a*
> *psychiatrist, and a coauthor of* The Beauty Prescription,
> *in Miami Beach, FL*

## RALLIE'S TIP

*My oldest son had colic. I'm sure this is the main reason that I waited 13 years to have another baby. I was young when I had my firstborn, and I hadn't yet been to medical school, so at the time I really had no idea that my baby was colicky. I just assumed that all babies cried a lot, rarely slept, and had projectile vomiting.*

*Like most moms, I tried everything that I could possibly think of to comfort my son. The one thing that helped the most was just holding him while I walked around or rocked him in a rocking chair. Sometimes it helped to put him in his car seat next to a running vacuum cleaner. How desperate does a mom have to be to think of trying something like that?!*

*Colic is as hard on parents as it is on their babies. It can lead to sleep deprivation, worry, and even despair. The only good thing about colic is that it eventually goes away. In the meantime, it's critical for moms and dads to take a break from their colicky babies when they're feeling overwhelmed. Ask someone you trust to watch your baby, even for an hour or two, and take some time to rest and regroup. And keep reminding yourself that this too shall pass.*

## Easing Colic

By definition, babies with colic are hard to console. It's not your imagination, and it's absolutely not you that's causing your baby's distress. Here are a few things that are worth a try to soothe him.

- White noise, such as the oven fan
- Movement, such as taking your baby for a walk
- Warmth, such as warm water bottle on his belly
- Distraction, such as giving your baby a bath
- Hold him with your hand under his stomach and his head on your forearm to put gentle pressure on his belly and relieve gas.

My daughter had horrible colic and reflux. We finally got that under control with Mylicon and oral Zantac.

—*Lisa M. Campanella-Coppo, MD, a mom of a six-year-old daughter and an emergency department physician at Summit Medical Group, in Livingston, NJ*

When my first baby had colic, what worked was holding her, walking around with her, and maybe rocking for a bit. I tried over-the-counter gas drops, but they didn't help. I honestly think they're more for the parents than the baby! My baby outgrew her colic by 8 weeks.

—*Aline T. Tanios Keyrouz, MD*

### Believe You Are the Best Mom

There are no medals in parenting. You don't earn stripes by surviving colic. But you should. In those really dark moments, when your baby is screaming and you feel like you don't have the strength to make it one more second, consider this: Maybe your baby was sent to you by God, the universe, whatever you believe, because wise, wonderful you are the absolute perfect mom for your baby. Only *you* are strong enough, caring enough, loving enough to do this. And do it, you will! You've got this! *You* are super, Mom.

My daughter had colic as a baby. To ease the crying, when my husband got home from work, he would walk her around. This gave me a break, but I couldn't listen to her cry, so I would put in earplugs or listen to music.

My baby's crying was so distressing for me. I swear it raised my blood pressure.

To try to calm my baby down, I would try to re-create the womb for her. I'd dim the lights, swaddle her tightly, run the vacuum cleaner for the shhhhh sound, and rock her gently from back to front. Babies are used to Mom walking, so rather than rocking them from side to side, rock them from back to front.

—*Eva Mayer, MD*

⁓

My older son was a tougher sleeper than my daughter. He had colic as an infant, which shaped how we responded to him. He cried often, and I felt like I didn't know how to read his signals well. I found myself in tears at times just trying to find the right way to soothe him, and I struggled with feeling unsuccessful and exhausted.

As first-time parents, we got a lot of advice from many different people. We were constantly trying to figure out the best way to take care of our first child. It was really hard, and I didn't have the opportunity to fully enjoy that newborn period with him because I was so caught up in getting it "right."

This experience really taught me a lot about making sure I follow my instincts about what my baby needs and what feels right for me. I think, on some level, my baby sensed our stress so that his crying and our stress became a self-perpetuating cycle.

Curiously, today my older son is one of the calmest and most reliably steady people I know. But he has times when he struggles with sleep, even now.

—*Sigrid Payne DaVeiga, MD, a mom of 10-year-old and 1-month-old sons and a 5-year-old daughter and a pediatric allergist with the Children's Hospital of Philadelphia, in Pennsylvania*

It was very difficult when my firstborn daughter had colic. I joked that if ob-gyns had return policies, their offices might be swamped with returned babies.

It's very difficult when your baby cries. Becoming a mother is supposed to be one of the happiest times of your life, and you feel so helpless when you can't comfort your own child. Moms with colicky babies often resort to ridiculous behaviors—jumping the babies around, rocking them for hours on end, and driving them in the car in circles. I finally resorted to putting my baby in her carseat and putting her on top of the running clothes dryer, supervised of course, which was in the laundry room down the hall from our apartment.

I traveled to Florida for a job interview and took my daughter with me. I hired a nurse to take care of her when I had to be away, and she told me that my breast milk was causing the colic. As a physician and mom, I thought that was ridiculous. But because I was at my wit's end, I tried not nursing her for 24 hours. My baby's colic came to a complete stop. Still not convinced, I reintroduced nursing. The crying started back up again, so once again I stopped nursing and my happy baby was back.

I was really upset about the whole situation. I went through a bit of a mourning period dealing with the decision not to nurse and the hormonal changes associated with it. But my baby was so much happier,

## When to Call Your Doctor: Colic

With as many as 40 percent of all babies experiencing colic, it can be hard to know when a crying jag is something you and your baby need to get through or if it's a warning sign that you need to call the doctor. Any time you suspect your baby's crying could be a sign of an illness, make the call. And certainly call your doctor immediately if your baby's temperature rises to 100.4°F or higher and if your infant is inconsolable for more than two hours, isn't eating, has diarrhea, is vomiting persistently, or is not as alert as usual, the Nemours Foundation says.

and I became so much happier having a baby I could manage without all the crying. We moved forward without nursing. My baby was only six weeks old at the time.

—*Eva Ritvo, MD*

ೕ൦

I have earned my PhD in colic. My first child, blessing though she was, was cursed with colic from day one. I was nursing. (At the time, I was working full-time in the military. If you've never tried to change out of chemical warfare gear to pump, you simply haven't lived!) I tried everything to get her to stop crying—from massage, to white noise, to dozens of special bottles, to Mylicon, to homeopathic tinctures. I would have tried just about anything if I thought there was any prayer of a good night's sleep.

My baby never slept anywhere except for on my chest, and she needed to be held perpetually. Thinking the warmth of my body soothed her, I tried warming her bed. It was to no avail.

I even tried putting my baby down on her tummy in stark violation of SIDS prevention rules—bad Mommy. But desperate times call for desperate measures. My husband would plead, "You're a doctor; you should know what to do!" I sobbed, "I have *no idea* what to do!"

We joked to our friends, after bailing out mid-dinner on too many occasions, that our daughter's middle name was "contraception."

Nothing ever worked. My baby eventually outgrew colic, though she didn't sleep through the night for 4+ years.

I truly blamed myself. I thought it was all my fault. However, when my twins came along 4½ years later, one of them had colic, but the other didn't. Hallelujah! I finally had proof that it wasn't my faulty parenting!

Little did I know, but that perfect breast milk I was dutifully feeding my kids caused significant allergic reactions in two of the three. The moment I stopped nursing the twins (at 3 months instead of 12 months for my first baby), the colic evaporated! Now I'm an expert in managing food sensitivities and healing the gut.

—*Susan Wilder, MD, a mom of a 22-year-old daughter and 17-year-old twins, a primary care physician, and the founder and CEO of LifeScape Premier, LLC, in Scottsdale, AZ*

## Mommy MD Guides–Recommended Product
### Colief Infant Digestive Aid

My baby cried so much. I felt that, as a physician, I should have known better what to do. I tried several products, and nothing helped. Then I heard about Colief Infant Digestive Aid.

The natural, dietary supplement drops worked great when my son was an infant. We were first time parents, and it was terrible to see our little guy in so much discomfort. We had tried other methods without much success. Colief drops were easy to administer and worked effectively. Now, I'm expecting my second child and feel assured that we are well prepared to deal with colic if it happens again, thanks to Colief.

—Arleen K. Lamba, MD, a mom of a three-year-old son, an anesthesiologist, the medical director of Blush Med Skincare, and founder of the Blush Blends Skin Care line, in Washington, DC

Colief Infant Digestive Aid is a gluten-free dietary supplement for the reduction of colic-associated crying resulting from temporary lactose intolerance (TLI) in infants. Different from other colic supplements, Colief Infant Digestive Aid is not given directly to the baby, but added to the formula or breast milk before each feeding, making it easier for them to digest the milk by breaking down most of the lactose.

If you're breastfeeding and your infant is experiencing colic, don't give up. It could be the lactose in the milk that's causing colic-associated crying, fussiness and gassiness because all breast milk naturally contains lactose. So if you suspect TLI is the cause of your infant's colic-associated crying, making major changes to your diet to eliminate certain foods while breastfeeding may not be necessary. Instead, try Colief Infant Digestive Aid, first, and see if TLI is the problem.

Colief is available at Walgreens for an average retail price of $19.95 or online at COLIEFUSA.COM. You can also visit their website to hear testimonials from other Colief moms.

*The maker of Colief is a paying partner of Momosa Publishing LLC. Regardless of whether we receive compensation from a vendor, we only recommend products or services that we have used personally and that we believe will be good for our readers.*

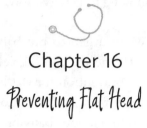

# Chapter 16
## Preventing Flat Head

If a baby develops a lasting flat spot, either on one side or the back of the head, it could be flat head syndrome, which is also called positional plagiocephaly (pu-ZI-shu-nul play-jee-oh-SEF-uh-lee). Flat head syndrome usually happens when a baby sleeps in the same position most of the time, or it can happen because of problems with a baby's neck muscles.

Premature babies are more likely to have flattened heads. Their skulls are softer than those of full-term babies. They also spend a lot of time on their backs without being moved or picked up because of their medical needs and extreme fragility after birth, which usually requires a stay in the neonatal intensive care unit (NICU).

### JUSTIFICATION FOR A CELEBRATION
When your baby can roll over, and you no longer have to worry so much about her developing a flat head, that should be a great reason to smile.

> **One in three healthy babies will develop some degree of flat head syndrome after birth. All babies are at risk. and it's even more common with multiple or premature births. But it's preventable.**
>
> *—Jane Scott, MD, pediatrician, neonatologist, and inventor of the Tortle repositioning beanie*

## Preventing Flat Head

Parenting is an ever-moving target! We solve one problem only to create another.

Case in point: We're urged to put babies to sleep on their backs, so they develop flat heads. Good grief.

Here's our favorite prevention for flat head: Hold your baby more! That's a pretty easy prescription to follow, right? Another prevention suggestion is to put your baby on her stomach as much as possible during the day while she's awake. Be sure to keep an eye on her so she doesn't fall asleep in this position.

Because babies are creatures of habit, they like to lie in the same position and look in the same direction. You need to mix it up for her. Place your baby in different positions in the crib, and move things around in her room to attraction her attention.

∽

My babies were held in arms so much during the day that I wasn't worried about their heads getting flattened.
—*Sharon Boyce, MD, a mom of seven- and five-year-old sons and a family physician with Oaklawn Medical Group in Albion and Bellevue, MI*

∽

My boys have always been very active. As babies, they spent a lot of time on their bellies, rolling around. Consequently, none of them developed a flat head.
—*Deborah Gilboa, MD, a mom of 14-, 12-, 10-, and 8-year-old sons, a family physician with Squirrel Hill Health Center, in Pittsburgh, PA, and a parenting speaker whose advice is found at AskDoctorG.com*

∽

To prevent flat head, we did a lot of tummy time during the day. This improved their coordination, and it also helped to tire baby out and prevent head flattening. Both are big plusses of tummy exercises!
—*Mona Gohara, MD, a mom of nine- and seven-year-old sons, a dermatologist in private practice, in Danbury, CT, and an associate clinical professor in the department of dermatology at Yale University*

Because we conformed to the "back to sleep" campaign, we had a flat-headed baby. But as our son started to do more tummy time, crawling, and rolling, that flat head resolved. He has a pretty perfect head now. Don't stress about the flat head; back to sleep is best.

—*Nilong Parikh Vyas, MD, MPH, a mom of seven- and five-year-old sons and the founder and owner of Sleepless in NOLA sleep consulting, in New Orleans, LA*

Because I always had my babies sleep on their backs, I worried about the rumors they would develop flat spots on their heads or not develop neck strength. I made sure they had lots of tummy time when they were awake. For example, I would put my baby on her stomach, and then I'd lie in front of her and play with finger puppets.

I did lots of silly things to keep her attention. This encouraged her to push up and strengthen her neck muscles. It's like a baby cobra yoga pose!

—*Lauren Hyman, MD, a mom of a 13-year-old daughter and an 11-year-old son and an ob-gyn at West Hills Hospital and Medical Center, in California*

### Get Glazed

If you have the two seconds to look at yourself in the mirror and comb your hair, have you noticed any grey? Shh, we promise not to tell anyone!

An inexpensive way to hide some grey hair and also increase your hair's shine is a glaze. Similar to a gloss, a hair glaze is temporary. Unlike a gloss, a glaze doesn't contain ammonia or peroxide, which are chemicals you don't want near yourself, let alone your baby!

Check out a salon like Hair Cuttery for a great glaze. It costs around $35. Visit **HAIRCUTTERY.COM** for more information.

When my daughters were babies, I made sure they had lots of tummy time, and I used a baby carrier to keep them upright. Despite all of those efforts, one of my daughters still developed a flatter area on her head. I think it's very hard to completely eliminate.

When my children were babies, it was recommended that babies sleep on their *stomachs*. Now, with babies sleeping on their backs, I think it's harder to prevent a flat head.

—*Kathryn Boling, MD, a mom of two grown daughters, a grandmom of two, and a family medicine physician with Mercy Medical Center, in Baltimore, MD*

Flat head can be fairly common. To prevent it, we rotated our babies' positions. One night , we put them down to sleep with their feet on one side of the crib, and the next night, we rotated them 180 degrees so their feet were on the other side.

This is effective because babies tend to focus on the same things most of the time. So if your baby is lying in the same position with the same objects to look at, her head may not move much. But by rotating her, the scenery changes, and her head moves in different positions, thus reducing the likelihood of a flat head.

*—Marcela Dominguez, MD, a mom of a 13-year-old daughter and an 11-year-old son who has a private family medicine and wellness practice in Southern California, whose concierge medicine services are provided by Signature MD*

We didn't really have much of a problem with flat heads. The key is to give babies a lot of tummy time and time upright. It wasn't something we were concerned about.

*—Leena S. Dev, MD, a mom of teenage boys and a general pediatrician, in Maryland*

## Treating Flat Head

The treatment for most cases of flat head is the same as prevention. In rare cases, a helmet might be prescribed. Never use a helmet without the direction of your baby's pediatrician. This

### Mommy MD Guides-Recommended Product
#### Tortle Head Repositioning Beanie

Jane Scott, MD, a mother of four and a pediatrician and neonatologist who lives in Colorado, created Tortle, a noninvasive affordable solution that treats mild cases and early diagnosed positional plagiocephaly (also known as flat head syndrome) in young infants. It can also prevent it from ever occurring. The Tortle is a patented, FDA-cleared device.

Tortle is a beanie that includes a support roll, which positions your baby's head in a way that helps prevent a flat head. You should reposition the support roll on the other side of your baby's head after two or three hours. Only use the beanie when you're supervising your baby while she sleeps, and don't use it overnight. An adjustable Tortle Head Repositioning beanie can be purchased for $24.99 at **TORTLE.COM.** You can also buy the beanies at retailers, including Target and Babies R Us.

treatment is used only in severe cases. Only a small percentage of babies wear helmets.

Generally babies have flat heads now. The only safe ways to prevent SIDS are no blankets, pillows, or stuffed animals in the crib, and sleeping on their backs. When babies grow up, their hair conceals the flat spot.

—*Larissa Guerrero, MD, a mom of a three-year-old son a nd family practice physician with Healthrow Ob/Gyn, in Orlando, FL*

## RALLIE'S TIP

*My firstborn was delivered with forceps, and he had a cone head for a couple of months after he was born. I remember how shocked I was when I saw his pointy little head for the first time! The pediatrician assured me that his head would be perfectly normal in time, and it was. So when my middle son started getting a flat spot on the back of his head, I wasn't too worried. I just started changing the position of his head slightly when I put him down to sleep, and the flat spot disappeared.*

### Mommy MD Guides-Recommended Product
#### Biddy Belly

When it's time for tummy time, try Biddy Belly, a cute giraffe your baby can lie on that's shaped specifically to help develop your baby's muscles during tummy time. The Biddy Belly positions your baby's arms correctly so she can push up, and the giraffe has a gradual incline to support your baby's weight and let her look around more easily. The Biddy Belly features a toy to keep her busy and happy, and it has bolsters to keep her from rolling off.

You can buy Biddy Belly online at **BIDDYBELLY.COM** or at specialty baby stores in Maryland and Kentucky for $39.99.

# Chapter 17
## *Solving Babies' Sleep Challenges*

So often in our parenting journeys, when we have a moment to think, Wow, things are going really well, the universe chuckles and throws us a new challenge. Daylight savings time, taking a vacation, having visitors, and colds and stomach bugs can derail even the best trips on the night train.

If your baby's sleep has been less than ideal, take heart in the fact that at least you're not a mama giraffe. They sleep only 1.9 hours a night. It could always be worse. Koalas, on the other hand, sleep 22 hours a day. But then koala bears aren't known for their high productivity.

### JUSTIFICATION FOR A CELEBRATION
We think the night that we turn the clocks back to gain an extra precious hour should be a mom holiday! Why not celebrate with a babysitter and an extra long date night?

> **Life's challenges are not supposed to paralyze you, they're supposed to help you discover who you are.**
>
> —*Bernice Johnson Reagon, singer and composer*

## Changing the Clocks

We urge you to do one very important thing when you're changing all of the clocks in your home—change your smoke detector batteries as well.

෨⁄෨

Any change in the routine caused havoc in my babies' sleep schedules. My strategy for daylight savings time was to move bedtime forward or backward (depending on the change) by 10- to 15-minute increments.

> *—Kathryn Boling, MD, a mom of two grown daughters, a grandmom of two, and a family medicine physician with Mercy Medical Center, in Baltimore, MD*

෨⁄෨

Any time there was a significant disruption in our lives, our babies' sleep schedule got disrupted. However, we tried to get back on track by making small adjustments, and we maintained flexibility if our schedules allowed. If we wanted to move their sleep time later, we would adjust it in 15-minute intervals.

For example, if we wanted the baby to sleep at 7:30 pm, and daylight savings time had just begun, we would allow four days to make the adjustment, in 15-minute increments each day. During the transition, we minimized disruptions. For example, we wouldn't plan any date nights.

> *—Edna Ma, MD, a mom of a 4-year-old son and an 18-month-old daughter, an anesthesiologist, and the founder of BareEASE pre-waxing numbing kit, in Los Angeles, CA*

෨⁄෨

Sometimes our babies got their days and nights mixed up! If they were having a hard time keeping day and night straight, during the day we would expose them to bright light to get their brains to recognize the light variation.

When my husband and I work a string of nights, we wear sunglasses during the day to prevent the light from keeping us awake. When we're trying to switch back to days, we get outside to get some sun to help kick our biological clocks back around to normal.

It's the same with our children. If their biological clocks seemed to be advancing toward falling asleep later at night and then waking up later in the morning, we would expose them to bright lights earlier in the day and then enforce bedtime at 6 pm.

*—Rebecca Jeanmonod, MD, a mom of 12- and 8-year-old daughters and 11- and 8-year-old sons and a professor of emergency medicine and the associate residency program director for the emergency medicine residency at St. Luke's University Health Network, in Bethlehem, PA*

When our children were babies, daylight savings time was rough. It really wreaked havoc on our sleep. You can establish a good routine and stick with it, but certain stresses and changes, like daylight savings time, are unavoidable.

I found it took a good week for my babies to adjust. The day after daylight savings time started didn't seem so bad. The second and third days were worse. After that it tapered off and then became the new normal.

*—Eva Ritvo, MD, a mom of two grown daughters, a psychiatrist, and a coauthor of* The Beauty Prescription, *in Miami Beach, FL*

### MomMy TIME — Enjoy that Day Light Savings Time Hour!

Your baby doesn't know it, but daylight savings time in the fall brings a precious extra hour of sleep. That likely means your child will be sleeping in an hour longer than usual, and you'll have another 60 minutes on your hands. Hurray! You might choose slumbering in your comfy bed, taking a relaxing bath instead of a five-minute shower, scrapbooking, crafting, putting together your child's memory book, or simply sipping your coffee while reading the newspaper or flipping through a magazine without interruption.

## BABY SLEEP PRO TIP: Tips for Time Changes

**Spring Forward.**

If your baby is a good sleeper on a good schedule, don't mess with it. Just wake her up at her usual time and put her to sleep the same time as always. It might take your baby a bit longer to fall asleep for a few days, but she'll adjust easily. Most good sleepers will adjust within a matter of days.

If you feel your baby isn't so adaptable or if you're worried about the change, plan ahead. If you prefer that your child adjusts by Sunday, when the time changes, start shifting your child's schedule on Tuesday or Wednesday. That means you need to schedule everything, even meals, 15 minutes earlier each day so that by Sunday your baby is ready to wake up at the usual wake time.

In other words, if your child usually awakens at 6:30 am, wake him at 6:15 am on Tuesday, 6 am on Wednesday, and so on. And if he usually naps at 12:30 pm, put him down at 12:15 pm Tuesday and 12 pm on Wednesday. And if bedtime is usually 6:30 pm, then shift to 6:15 pm, and then 6 pm, and finally to 5:45 pm until you have shifted the entire schedule one hour earlier. By Sunday, when you move the clocks one hour ahead, your baby will be waking up and going to bed at the usual times.

With either technique, the following tips will help make the time change easier on everyone:

**Make it dark.** Although everyone loves longer days, it can still be quite bright at bedtime, which makes it harder to fall asleep. Install room darkening shades to help the transition to sleep.

**Expose to light!** Exposing your child to bright light early in the morning and dimmer light later in the day helps reset the circadian rhythm, or daily internal clock, which is regulated by light and dark.

**Fall Back.**

If your baby is a good sleeper on a good schedule, do nothing. Kids who are well rested, adaptable, and on predictable sleep schedules will adjust to the new time easily over the course of a couple days. The key is to move to the new time as quickly as possible while respecting their sleep cues that might indicate they are tired a little earlier than usual. Remember they may wake earlier for a few days. For example, if they usually wake at 6:30 am, they may wake at 5:30 am at first. But encourage your baby to stay in bed a little longer so that his clock can reset. An early wake up may mean that he may be tired earlier for naps and bedtime. Respect that and don't push him to the point of becoming overtired. Maybe naps and bedtime will occur 30 minutes earlier for a couple days while adjusting to the new time.

If your baby isn't such a good sleeper or if you're worried about the change, start early. Three to four days before the time change, shift your baby's entire daily schedule later in 15-minute intervals. That includes meals, naps, activities, and bedtimes.

So if your child usually naps at 9 am and 1 pm, then shift the nap to 9:15 am and 1:15 pm the first day and then 9:30 am and 1:30 pm the next, and so on. By Sunday, he will be fully adjusted. The same goes for meals, activities, and bedtimes. This will allow your baby's biological clock to adjust over the course of a few days.

With either technique, the following three tips will make resetting the clock a little easier on everyone.

**Make it dark.** Because it will be lighter earlier in the morning, remember to make your child's room as dark as possible to increase the chances she will stay asleep. Darkness increases melatonin production, while light reduces it.

**Get outside!** Exposure to bright light in the late afternoon can help make the transition to a later bedtime easier.

**Watch for sleepy cues.** If your child usually goes to bed at 7 pm, she may be tired by 6 pm for a couple nights after the clocks change. Watch for sleep cues and avoid the dreaded overtired meltdown by getting her in bed earlier for a few days while her internal clock gradually shifts to the new time. The same holds true for naps.

Using these sleep strategies, most kids will adjust to the new time within a week if not sooner.

—**Rebecca Kempton, MD**

## Traveling and Vacations

Some things are worth a little inconvenience and lack of sleep. A trip—Walt Disney World anyone?—falls into that category!

～⌒

One of the best things about our bedtime routine was that it was completely portable. It didn't matter if we were home, on vacation, or at overnight camp. Our routine was always the same. When we pulled out two storybooks, said a prayer, and sang two songs, my boys knew it was time for bed.

*—Deborah Gilboa, MD, a mom of 14-, 12-, 10-, and 8-year-old sons, a family physician with Squirrel Hill Health Center, in Pittsburgh, PA, and a parenting speaker whose advice is found at AskDoctorG.com*

～⌒

Having a bedtime ritual that was largely the same every night helped when we traveled. We kept as close to our usual routine as possible wherever we were. We sang the same songs and tried to stick with regular mealtimes and our sleep schedule.

When we traveled, we took our white noise machine and our daughter's special lovey. Now, smartphones make it easier to always have white noise. You can find white noise apps on the app store.

*—Katja Rowell, MD, a mom of a 10-year-old daughter, a family practice physician, and the author of* Helping Your Child with Extreme Picky Eating and Love Me, Feed Me *at TheFeedingDoctor.com, in St. Paul, MN*

～⌒

For bigger changes to the routine, such as a vacation that included a time change, we tried to arrive at our destination early in the day and keep our daughters awake as much as possible during the daytime hours. We hoped this would help them to sleep well the first night and adjust quickly to the time change.

*—Kathryn Boling, MD*

～⌒

We found that vacations and visitors wrecked our babies' sleep, and they still do today although our kids are now five and three years old!

The thing that kept my husband and me from panicking was that we always knew it was just a matter of a day or two to get back on schedule. We believed that having visitors and taking vacations were worth a night or two of less-than-ideal sleep for our kids and us.

The need to get back on track was always just a temporary problem. To get back on track, we just went back to our previous schedule, and things fell into place.

—*Jennifer Bacani McKenney, MD, a mom a five-year-old daughter and a three-year-old son and a family physician, in Fredonia, KS*

⌒⌒

Travel was difficult with babies, especially when we crossed time zones. Some babies thrive in different environments and sleep fine. Others don't like it, and the change throws them off entirely.

When we traveled, I tried to keep my babies' sleep routine similar to what we did at home. I brought their sleep blankets, stuffed animals, and favorite books. It's helpful for children to have something familiar with them from home.

I used to joke that we went on "trips," not "vacations," because we never knew how it was going to go. Sometimes it went well, and it felt like a vacation. Other times, it was merely a trip. It helps to have realistic expectations.

At the end of the day, travel is going to disrupt your routine. There's really no way around it. Choose your trips wisely!

—*Eva Ritvo, MD*

⌒⌒

When we went on vacation, my husband and I wanted to spend some time alone too. We would feed our babies dinner by 6 pm and put them to bed. Then we'd order delivery from the hotel restaurant and sit on the balcony, leaving the balcony door cracked open so we could hear our kids if they needed us. This gave us a little space—and privacy!

—*Marcela Dominguez, MD, a mom of a 13-year-old daughter and an 11-year-old son who has a private family medicine and wellness practice in Southern California, whose concierge medicine services are provided by Signature MD*

## BABY SLEEP PRO TIP: Travel Tips

Here are my top tips to help your baby—and you —sleep well on a trip.

**Start your trip well rested.** Travel—whether by car, plane, or train—can rob anyone of shut eye, but it especially takes its toll on young children and babies, who accumulate sleep debts quickly. Aim to have your child well rested before leaving on your trip, taking restorative naps and sleeping well at night for the days preceding your departure. Babies and children whose sleep tanks are full can adapt much easier to schedule changes and a little lost sleep here or there.

**Plan travel time around sleep time.** Because children are naturally excited or even stimulated by travel plans, it's often hard for them to sleep en route. Try to plan your departure and arrival times around naps as much as possible. If your child still naps in the morning, plan to leave after the morning nap, not before. The first nap is usually the most restorative and helps curb overtiredness for the rest of the day. Also, transit naps are never as restful as naps at home. As much as possible, try to arrive at your destination in time for the usual bedtime. If the naps were shorter than usual, aim for an earlier bedtime.

**Think ahead about sleeping conditions.** Going from having their own bedrooms to crowding everyone into one bedroom can spell disaster for everyone's sleep. If you plan to stay in a hotel, splurge on a suite to give you some extra living space with a pull-out bed or a crib. This will allow you to enjoy the evening while your little ones sleep nearby; it may even save you on food expenses if you also have a kitchenette to store your own milk and snacks. Finding a condo or private home has become easier than ever with sites like vrbo.com and airbnb.com. Extra sleeping space makes for a more relaxed vacation for everyone.

If you're in a single hotel room, all is not lost! Get creative and think about where you can put a crib or small bed that's separate from your bed. Sometimes it may mean putting the crib in the bathroom, a hallway, or even a large closet. Rearranging the furniture can help. Or try to hang a sheet from the ceiling to create a physical separator.

Hotel staff members are usually more than willing to help you "redecorate" in the name of sleep.

All is not lost if your toddler ends up in your bed even though it isn't your ideal sleeping arrangement. The key to a successful transition back home is communication ahead of time. Tell your child this is a special sleeping arrangement just for the trip. When you return, you'll be back in your own bed, and he will be in his. Frequent reminders about sleep rules, even on the trip home, are important to avoid the temptation to join you in bed upon your return.

**Buy, rent, or reserve the beds you'll need.** If you stay with family on a regular basis, buy, ask family members to borrow, or rent a portable crib. If you're staying in a hotel, call in advance, so the cribs or extra pull-out beds will be ready when you check in. If you're traveling by car, bring your own bed (BYOB). A Pack 'n Play or travel bed or sleeping bags for older kids are great portable options that you'll use many times.

**Do practice runs.** Trips cause a lot of disruptions to familiar routines, whether it's at a hotel or your in-law's house. You don't want to arrive only to have your child go into meltdown mode. If you take your own travel bed or portable crib, allow your child to sleep in it a few nights before you leave to get used to it. Also, prior to departure, talk with toddlers about new sleeping arrangements and any additional plans.

**Take along helpful sleep accessories.** Have you ever packed a suitcase full of toys only to never unzip the bag? I have! But these days I've exchanged the extra toy bag for one with some helpful sleep accessories. Here are some lightweight and useful options.

• **White noise app:** Download a white noise app, such as "Relax Melodies." White noise is extremely soothing for babies and toddlers, and it can help drown out ambient noise, which may be unavoidable away from home.

• **A favorite stuffed animal or loveys:** Bring one or two portable stuffed animals, loveys, or dolls your child won't sleep without. But not a whole menagerie!

_ZZZZz_

## BABY SLEEP PRO TIP: Travel Tips _(continued)_

• **Sheets:** Even when traveling without the crib, consider taking your own sheets. The familiar patterns, the texture, and smell can help a child transition to a new sleeping environment. Hotels (or even family) may not have appropriately-sized sheets, so it's better to take along your own.

• **Black plastic bags and some painter's tape:** They won't win any design awards, but garbage bags make great black out "curtains" in a pinch and can help create darkness that's essential for melatonin release and sleep.

• **Strollers:** With travel more challenging than ever, expect delays. Even toddlers old enough to walk easily may benefit from rest on wheels, especially at an airport when there are flight delays. Pushing a stroller is a whole lot easier than giving shoulder rides through the airport or amusement parks.

**Re-create bedtime routines.** Despite changes in schedules and scenery, try to keep bedtime routines constant. If bath, books, and song are parts of your normal routine, stick to them. If Grandma or Uncle Bob want to participate, let them join in or take over! It's not so much about who does it, but that the routines are as consistent and predictable as they are at home.

**Squeeze in naps as much as possible.** Whether walking through Disney World or spending time with your family, it's tempting to eliminate the nap while on vacation. Skipping routine naps spells trouble! If your schedule necessitates a skipped nap one day, try to plan a lighter schedule the next day to allow for crucial daytime rest. If you do miss a nap, compensate with an earlier bedtime. The more the sleep deficit accumulates, the greater the risk of the dreaded meltdown—even if you're at the zoo! Be flexible, but accommodate the daytime sleep needs as much as possible, even if it means napping in the stroller or air-conditioned car or at the beach. When your child naps, take advantage of a midday siesta yourself! It's a great fix for the whole family.

**Anticipate time differences.** If you're traveling across time zones, it's best to move your schedule to the new time zone as soon as possible. Allow a few days to get sleep back on track both when arriving or returning home. If you're only traveling for two to four days across one or two time zones, it's sometimes easiest to stay on your home time zone. If you're traveling for a longer period to a different time zone, consider shifting to the new time zone the week before your travel. Modify your children's sleeping and eating routines 15 minutes earlier, or later, each day prior to the trip. This may take three to four days, so plan ahead.

If you don't make the adjustments prior to leaving, aim to shift your child to the new time zone as soon as you arrive. So you could wake your child as close as possible to his regular wake up time on the the new time zone. Or you could allow hime to wake up early and put him to bed at the usual time in the new time zone. The same goes for naps. Expose your child to bright light early in the morning and dim light in the early evening if you're traveling east, and do the opposite traveling west. This helps shift your child's circadian rhythms and makes the transition easier.

**Break some rules and have fun!** Try not to stress about strict sleep habits on vacation. Kids are surprisingly resilient. If they miss a few naps and go to bed too late a few nights, they'll survive and so will you! Let kids have fun doing something they don't usually do. If you disturb a few people—fellow passengers or other hotel visitors—along the way, you won't see them again, so don't worry!

**Get back on track as soon as you get home.** Sometimes the hardest part of a trip is resuming normal routines when you return. Staying up late eating popcorn at Grandma's is so much more fun than hitting the hay at 7 pm every night. Don't bring vacation habits home with you. Try to get back to nap and bedtime routines as soon as possible, knowing that it might take a few days and a few tears to get back on track.

—*Rebecca Kempton, MD*

## Coping with Illnesses

A sick baby might be a sleepy baby. Or not.

The greatest challenge to our baby sleeping was when he was sick. Those nights, he slept on my chest in a recliner in his bedroom.

—*Larissa Guerrero, MD, a mom of a three-year-old son and family practice physician with Healthrow Ob/Gyn, in Orlando, FL*

I found that my babies slept more when they were sick, not less. The only challenge was that when they were sick, they'd want to crawl into bed with me. If I was really tired, I'd let them get away with it. But usually, they slept off the illness in their own rooms.

—*Sharon Boyce, MD, a mom of seven- and five-year-old sons and a family physician with Oaklawn Medical Group, in Albion and Bellevue, MI*

Our daughter had gastroesophageal reflux disease (GERD) when she was a baby. If your baby has GERD, it helps to elevate her head, but there's not really a practical or safe way to do this. For the most part, it helps to feed your baby as far ahead of time before bed as possible and to talk with your doctor about medications.

—*Lisa M. Campanella-Coppo, MD, a mom of a six-year-old daughter and an emergency department physician at Summit Medical Group, in Livingston, NJ*

The first few months after my daughter started day care were complicated by illness because she was exposed to all the germs at day care. Colds and coughs made for more restless nights. It was a hard time of adjustment for all of us.

—*Kathryn Boling, MD*

My babies didn't get sick often. I attribute that to breastfeeding and implementing good sleep habits from the beginning.

When my babies did get colds, I used a bulb suction device to clear the mucus from their noses. To do this correctly, you flatten the

**MomMy TIME**

### Sip Chamomile Tea

Sipping a tea made from the herb chamomile can help reduce anxiety and make it easier to wind down at the end of the day and prepare for bed. Take a few minutes to indulge in a cup in the evenings.

bulb, put the tip in the baby's nose, and release the bulb. Discard any mucous in the sink by squeezing and releasing the bulb several times. Do this in each nostril if needed.

When I was done using the bulb, I would clean the tip with soap and water, then rub it with alcohol and air dry it.

I also gave my children steam treatments. I'd simply have them sit in the bathroom while someone else was taking a shower. This helped them to breathe—and sleep—better.

If our babies were really sick, such as with a stomach virus, my husband and I took turns being "on call" for them at night. We would wake up with them, check a rectal temperature if needed, and rock them back to sleep.

—*Marcela Dominguez, MD*

When my kids were sick, it upset their sleep. My husband and I worried about them. But we never let them sleep in our bed.

We didn't want to set that precedent. With two working parents, it was critical that at least one of us got a good night's sleep—sleeping in our own bed. Instead, when they were sick, such as with a cold or stomach virus, we slept in their rooms with them. Usually, we'd cuddle them up in their beds, but sometimes we ended up wrapped in blankets on the floor.

—*Lauren Hyman, MD, a mom of a 13-year-old daughter and an 11-year-old son and an ob-gyn at West Hills Hospital and Medical Center, in California*

> **A good laugh and a long sleep are
> the best cures in the doctor's book.**
> —**Irish Proverb**

I remember when my son got a GI bug as an infant. He threw up multiple times. We got him up and out of his wet, vomit-soaked crib, (he was smiling). We gave him some Pedialyte, changed his sheets, and laid him back down. He went back to sleep. My husband and I were shocked.

Once we skipped my son's nap to take him to a parade. He wasn't used to skipping naps. When he got home, he was acting very sleepy, so we put him down; it was 4 pm He slept the entire night and woke up the next day at 7 am! He didn't wake once!

Because my kids were so set in their schedules and so well caught up on sleep, when a tooth would erupt or when they had an illness, we wouldn't sometimes know about it until the next morning because they didn't wake up in the middle of the night. I remember going to a well-child visit with my son, and the doctor said, "He has three molars coming out at the same time." I said, "Oh, I didn't even know; he's been sleeping fine."

I think teething gets blamed for a lot of sleep issues, as does travel, illness, and daylight savings time. But if you stay consistent and your kids get the sleep they need, occasional disturbances don't typically affect their overall sleep patterns.

Consistency is the key to good sleep. Also, kids can fight infections better if they're better rested. Some parents say, "My kid slept for three hours today!" Well, if they're sick, that's what they're supposed to do to heal themselves.

## Mommy MD Guides–Recommended Product
### HoMedics Sound Machine

For both children, we used the HoMedics sound machine for white noise. It's great because it stays on all night, it can be plugged in or can run on batteries, it's small enough to take on trips, it has options for different sounds, and it's reasonably priced at around $20.
—Jennifer Bacani McKenney, MD

*—Nilong Parikh Vyas, MD, MPH, a mom of seven- and five-year-old sons and the founder and owner of Sleepless in NOLA sleep consulting, in New Orleans, LA*

## Mommy MD Guides-Recommended Product
### Rallie's Tip-Winix HR1000

Because indoor air quality can be worse than the air outside, it's important to do all that you can to purify the air that your family breathes.

I love the Winix HR1000. My air actually smells purer, if that's possible, and it's a great source of white noise. Plus it's very classy looking. I put it right in my living room, where I can admire it and breathe wonderful pure air!

Ironically, the air inside your home might not be the best air for you and your family to breathe. According to the U.S. Consumer Product Safety Commission, research has shown that the air inside our homes might be more polluted than the air outside— even the air in the largest, most industrialized cities.

According to the American Environmental Protection Agency, indoor air pollution is one of the top five health threats today. Breathing polluted air can lead to health effects, ranging from worsening allergies and asthma to cardiovascular problems.

Winix, the leader in healthy home appliance technology, offers the HR1000, one of the first wi-fi enabled air purifiers on the market that works from your smart phone or tablet. When the air purifier is paired with the Winix Smart app, you can control the unit from anywhere and track your home's indoor air quality as well as the outdoor air. This information empowers you to make changes, if necessary, to lead a healthier lifestyle.

You can buy a Winix HR1000 at stores, such as Home Depot, for around $380. Visit **WINIXAMERICA.COM** for more information.

## Easing Separation Anxiety and Other Sleep Challenges

In so many cultures, babies, mommies, grandmommies, and the cat all sleep together. Some days, we really see the wisdom in that.

My daughter would cry when I went to work. Fifteen minutes later, my nanny would text me pictures of my daughter playing happily. Meanwhile, I'm sobbing on my drive in to work. I think my daughter's separation anxiety was shorter-lived than mine. I don't think her separation anxiety impacted her sleep because she didn't go down for a nap until hours after I left for work, which was a good strategy.

—*Lisa M. Campanella-Coppo, MD*

*All* babies have sleep challenges at some point. The best advice I have is that whatever is now will not always be. Try to remember that, especially when you're tired and frustrated. When your baby isn't sleeping, it's easy to convince yourself that he will *never* sleep. You might worry he'll never go to college, let alone overnight camp, because he's never going to sleep. I promise that your child *will* sleep.

The secret to good parenting is to remember that almost everything is a phase—the good and the bad. Everything changes—not just sleep. Everything that you are dealing with now will be different in two months. Try not to drive yourself bananas.

With my first baby, I tried everything to get him to sleep. I remember times when he was extremely cranky because he was so tired. I thought, *You are so tired! Just go to sleep!*

Sometimes, babies get so overwhelmed by stimuli that they can't fall asleep. Then they get *overtired*. One time, my husband literally put his hand over our baby's eyes to block everything out. He held his hands there for a few moments, and the baby fell asleep.

—*Deborah Gilboa, MD*

## RALLIE'S TIP

*When my youngest two children were babies, I was a medical resident and my husband was an emergency physician. I had to work nights at the hospital three times a week, and my husband worked night shifts one* week out of every month. My children were accustomed to having only one parent present at bedtime some evenings, and usually it didn't bother them. But sometimes, especially when they were overtired or not feeling well, they would get a little anxious about the working parent, and that would make it difficult for them to get to sleep.

We tried having a goodnight phone call with the working parent, but that was a big mistake! We thought it would be comforting, but it actually highlighted the fact that someone was missing.

My husband and I worked hard to keep the bedtime ritual consistent whether one or both of us were at home, and I think that was important in keeping separation anxiety to a minimum. The home parent gave the boys their baths, then snuggled and read books, and then said goodnight. If one or both of my sons needed a little extra cuddling or reassurance to relax and go to sleep, that was fine.

Separation anxiety is practically inevitable when young children are away from their parents, especially at bedtime, but most of us just can't be with our children 24/7. The best we can do is keep things as consistent as possible when we have to be away. Following the normal routine is comforting and reassuring, and it makes it easier for children to deal with the absence of a parent at bedtime.

## ? When to Call Your Doctor: Separation Anxiety

Separation anxiety moves from being a normal part of a child's development to a psychological disorder when your child starts becoming highly distressed.

If your baby is extremely anxious about being separated and believes something bad will happen when you're separated, it may be a sign of separation anxiety disorder. Your child may also complain of physical symptoms, such as a headache, stomachache, or dizziness in anticipation of being separated. If this is the case, call your doctor. Your child may need therapy, with which he'll learn how to deal with his fears.

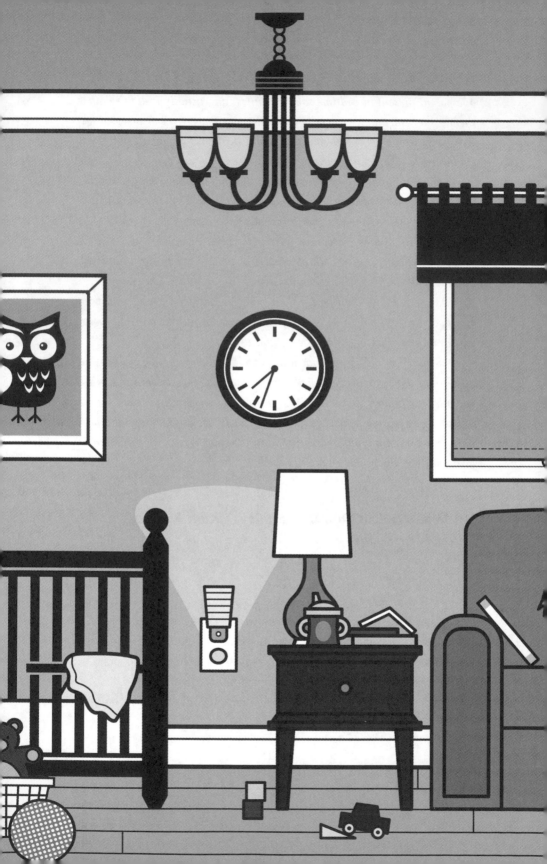

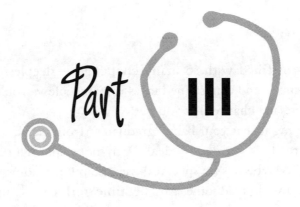

# TODDLERS: 1 YEAR TO 3 YEARS

# Chapter 18

## Transitioning to a Toddler Bed

Parenting is filled with so many challenges—sleepless nights, skinned knees, and tear-stained faces to name a few. You deserve to celebrate any chance that you get!

The night that your baby "graduates" from a crib to a toddler bed really is a really big deal. Why not make it a reason to celebrate? Maybe bake a special dessert, blow out some candles and make a wish, read some extra bedtime stories, make up a new sleepytime song—whatever makes you and your little one smile.

Your toddler will only get to transition from a crib to a toddler bed one time, after all. Why not make it memorable?

### JUSTIFICATION FOR A CELEBRATION

It's a good bet you'll feel a twinge of sadness when your toddler moves from the crib to a bed. But really it's a cause celeb instead!

> **O bed! O bed! delicious bed!**
> **That heaven upon earth to the weary head.**
>
> —*Thomas Hood,* Miss Kilmansegg—Her Dream

## Timing the Transition

Especially if your little one has had sleep challenges, you're probably concerned that such a big change of going from a crib to a bed is going to wreck her sleep yet again. Timing is *everything*.

&#x2053;

Each of my kids transitioned to a bed at or slightly before age two. It was mainly because the next child was waiting in the wings and needed a crib. My kids (all six of them) are two years or less apart.

—*Susan Besser, MD, a mom of six grown children, a grandmom of five, and a family physician at River Family Physicians, in Easton, MD*

&#x2053;

When our kids were four and five years old, we transitioned them to toddler beds. We put a nightlight in the room so they could see.

—*Shilpa Amin-Shah, MD, a mom of a 6-year-old son and 5-year-old and 18-month-old daughters and an emergency medicine physician at Emergency Medical Associates, in St. Johns, FL*

&#x2053;

We transitioned our daughter to a toddler bed when she was two years old. It actually was a challenge because she's a very active sleeper and needed more room to move around. The smaller toddler bed led to her waking up more than she had in her crib.

—*Lisa M. Campanella-Coppo, MD, a mom of a six-year-old daughter and an emergency department physician at Summit Medical Group, in Livingston, NJ*

&#x2053;

When my daughter had to give up her crib for the expected arrival of my son, we did the transition in stages over a few months. First, we moved the crib mattress to the floor, and we moved the crib itself out of the room.

After a few weeks of my daughter sleeping on the crib mattress on the floor, we replaced it with a larger twin-size mattress, still on the floor. Finally, a few months later, my daughter's big-girl bed arrived, and the mattress she was already comfortable sleeping on was moved up into the frame. The slow transition worked beautifully!

When it was time for my son to leave the crib, we again put the mattress on the floor, and we transitioned him to a bed the same way.

—*Lauren Hyman, MD, a mom of a 13-year-old daughter and 11-year-old son and an ob/gyn in at West Hills Hospital and Medical Center, in California*

❧

I always advise waiting as long as possible to make the transition from crib to bed because it can be a tricky one if done too early. We waited until my son was three years old.

Before age three, children don't understand imaginary boundaries, and they have only a preliminary notion of consequences of their behaviors. Because of that, when we move them to a bed too early, it can be extremely challenging to actually keep them there because they are more keen to test their new-found independence than to follow the rules of staying in bed.

—*Rebecca Kempton, MD, a mom of eight- and six-year-old sons and a three-year-old daughter and an infant and toddler sleep specialist, in Chicago, IL*

❧

We transitioned each of my kids to a toddler bed when they were around two years old. That's when they started to become too big for the crib, climbing out of it, sometimes having their legs stuck between the crib rails.

Before my son was born, I needed the crib that my oldest daughter was still sleeping in! I started to transition her out of it two months before her brother was born to minimize the feeling that she was being displaced.

—*Aline T. Tanios Keyrouz, MD, a mom of 13- and 7-year-old and 9-month-old daughters and an 11-year-son and an assistant professor of pediatrics at St. Louis University, in Missouri*

❧

I think parents take their kids out of the crib way too soon, and it ends up leading to more sleep difficulties because a two-year-old cannot understand rewards and consequences and will take advantage of the new-found freedom of getting in and out of a toddler bed. Children typically don't understand rewards and consequences at 18 months or even two years of age. But by 2½ and four years old, they definitely can.

My rule is, once a baby is nighttime potty trained, he's moved into a toddler bed so he can get up to urinate, if needed. We kept my older son in his crib in his room until he was nighttime potty trained (at four years of age), and then he moved into a toddler bed in his room.

—*Nilong Parikh Vyas, MD, MPH, a mom of seven- and five-year-old sons and the founder and owner of Sleepless in NOLA sleep consulting, in New Orleans, LA*

༄

Soon after we found out we were expecting our son, my husband and I transitioned our daughter to a big girl bed. She was about two years old. We wanted to give her time before our son was born to get used to the idea of a bigger bed.

We still haven't transitioned my son, who only recently turned three, because he loves his crib. We're planning on buying either bunk beds or at least bigger beds for them both, which will likely help with our storytime-before-bed routine.

—*Manpreet K. Gill, MD, a mom of a five-year-old daughter and a three-year-old son and a family practice physician with North Seminole Family Practice, in Sanford, FL*

༄

I may not be the best parent to ask about transitioning to a toddler bed! Our four-year-old toddler still sleeps in the master bed with me! My philosophy is that since the dawn of time, parents have slept with their children and provided them with comfort and security. Toddler beds are a modern invention for the convenience of parents.

There's nothing wrong with using toddler beds! But for me, I feel this phase in our lives, while my children are still young and want to sleep next to me, is fleeting.

In a few years, when my son is ready, he will no longer want to cuddle with me. But for now, we both enjoy sleeping next to each other at night.

—*Edna Ma, MD, Transitioning to a Toddler Bedth-old daughter, an anesthesiologist, and the founder of BareEASE pre-waxing numbing kit, in Los Angeles, CA*

## BABY SLEEP PRO TIP
### Crib-to-Bed Transition Dos and Don'ts

**Do time it right.** Wait as long as possible to make the transition, preferably until your child is at least three years old. Why? Children under age three have difficulty understanding boundaries that are not physical, like the bars of a crib. Therefore, the transition to a bed, if done too early, can result in night wakings and night wanderings, which can be scary, hard to prevent, and even dangerous.

**Don't use your child's nimble crib escape** as a reason to transition to a bed. Try these tips first!

• Put a sleep sack on your baby to make it more difficult for her to scale the crib.

• Turn the crib around: If your crib has one side that is higher, turn it so the high side faces out and the low side is against a wall. This can make it difficult for even for the most agile climbers to escape.

• Lower the mattress to the ground, even below the lowest setting. This can make it impossible to climb over even for tall toddlers.

• Use a video monitor to catch your child in the act of climbing. Go into the room (or talk through the monitor) as they are climbing out and sternly say "No!" This method is extremely effective if you can catch your child in the act, but you might need to repeat several times.

**Do establish sleep rules.** Have fun making a poster that your child can decorate. Outline the rules (with pictures) of the big kid bed and the importance of staying in it for the whole night so she can get the sleep she needs.

**Do have a plan if your child escapes!** Return your child to bed silently and consistently so the behavior is not rewarded.

**Do make your child's room safe.** Ensure furniture is attached to the wall and there's nothing she can hurt herself with because she can now roam freely. Toddler bed rails can help as well.

—*Rebecca Kempton, MD*

## Choosing a Bed

Bed shopping is fun! Bring your toddler along and make it special!

∽

I didn't purchase a toddler bed. My children slept in cribs until they were about two or three. Then they slept in regular single beds.

*—Elizabeth Berger, MD, a mom of two grown children, a child psychiatrist, and the author of* Raising Kids with Character, *in New York City*

∽

When we transitioned my older son to a toddler bed—because we had another baby coming—we were on a small budget. We purchased a decent toddler bed from a department store. It lasted us through two toddlers, so it worked out just fine.

*—Leena S. Dev, MD, a mom of teenage boys and a general pediatrician, in Maryland*

∽

Initially, we put our children in a twin platform bed with side rails. We used Summer infant brand and found it very easy to assemble.

When our first two kids were four and five years old, we moved to a new house. We got toddler beds from Babies R Us brand, which I recommend for the price and fact that we only used them for one year. We found their small size and short distance from the ground comforting for the children.

I placed soft blankets next to the beds in case my kids rolled out. We also continued to use the video monitor.

*—Shilpa Amin-Shah, MD*

∽

My daughter didn't sleep well in a toddler bed. It was too small. She needed more room to move around. We switched her to a regular twin bed with side rails when she was three years old. She slept much better in the bigger bed!

*—Lisa M. Campanella-Coppo, MD*

∽

When our son was transitioning to the crib at six weeks old, we transitioned our nearly two-year-old daughter to a bed. She actually slept in the middle of a queen-sized bed that was in the bedroom next to ours. Either my mom or I slept with her at first to make sure she could sleep there. She did fine.

Once my daughter was able to sleep alone, we installed railings along all open sides of her bed to prevent her from falling out. She slept in a cotton onesie with a sheet and quilted comforter.

—*Marcela Dominguez, MD, a mom of a 13-year-old daughter and an 11-year-old son who has a private family medicine and wellness practice in Southern California, whose concierge medicine services are provided by Signature MD*

## Making the New Bed Special

Change is hard for most of us, especially for most toddlers. It's hard not to be sad about what you're giving up. The secret is to be *happier* about what you're getting. That makes the loss easier to bear. It's helpful to let your child be sad about giving up the crib, if that's her nature. But try to focus on the positive, the new bed she's getting, rather than the old crib she's leaving behind.

⌒⌒

My oldest daughter slept in a bed just before she turned three years old. We made a big deal about her being a big girl now and how she had a newborn baby sister who slept in the crib, where babies sleep. My older daughter was ready for the transition, and she adjusted almost immediately.

—*Kathryn Boling, MD, a mom of two grown daughters, a grandmom of two, and a family medicine physician with Mercy Medical Center, in Baltimore, MD*

To help entice my daughter to sleep in her own bed, we told her from the beginning that her bed was the most comfortable bed in the house!

—*Lauren Hyman, MD*

When I transitioned each of my kids from the crib to a bed, I tried to make the change special. I wanted them to feel like they were graduating from being a baby in a crib to a toddler in a bed.

I took each of my kids shopping. I let them each pick out some new bedding with their favorite cartoon characters on it.

—*Aline T. Tanios Keyrouz, MD*

When my son was three years old, we transitioned him to a toddler bed. We made a big deal about the big boy bed—letting him pick out fun sheets and a new stuffed animal to make the occasion special. We also made a big poster of bedtime rules to make sure he understood that having a big boy bed meant he also had to follow the rules around sleep time and stay in it!

—*Rebecca Kempton, MD, a mom of eight- and six-year-old sons and a three-year-old daughter and an infant and toddler sleep specialist, in Chicago, IL*

### Taking Those Last Nursery Photos

There's much excitement surrounding the arrival of the toddler bed. It's an exciting transition for your toddler, and it's also an emotional milestone for you. Take some time to honor those feelings.

Don't let the anticipation make you forget to snap some last pictures of your child's room before you take down the crib rails. Your baby is growing up, and you'll be happy you preserved those memories of her nursery as it was during the first couple of years of her life.

## BABY SLEEP PRO TIP: Celebrate Transitions

When your toddler is ready to transition to a big kid bed, make a big deal about it. Use the transition as a reward for great sleep habits when the time is right. Take your child to the store to choose a bed and some new sheets and even a new stuffed animal to snuggle with in her new bed.

—*Rebecca Kempton, MD*

## Mommy MD Guides–Recommended Product
### Step2 Hot Wheels Toddler-to-Twin Bed, Thomas & Friends Toddler Bed, and Princess Palace Bed

Your little one can race all day and night with the Hot Wheels Toddler-to-Twin Bed from Step 2. It looks like a Hot Wheels car, complete with a place to show off his Hot Wheels collection on the air intakes and spoiler. This kid's car bed makes the transition from a crib easy and fun. It grows with your child as it transforms into a twin bed. The bed costs $299.99–$349.99.

If your little one is more of a train fan, the Step2 Thomas & Friends Toddler Bed means he can chug-chug-chug all night with his favorite friend. Thomas' smoke stack has special storage for your child's bedtime books. It costs $169.99–$199.99.

For little princesses, Step 2 has a Princess Palace Twin Bed. The bed features a headboard with twin towers, "windows" with a scenic "view outside of the castle." Spaces on the "window sills" are perfect for alarm clock, books and more. Protective, wide side rails accommodate you to sit on for story time. It has a built-in light. The beds cost $320.00–$349.99.

You can buy all of these beds at **ToyRUs.com, Amazon.com, Walmart.com,** and **Step2.com.**

# Chapter 19

## Toddler Napping

Only 15 percent of mammals, including people, are monophasic sleepers. That means we sleep for a long stretch of time, then we're awake for a long stretch.

The other 85 percent of mammals, including cats and new-born babies, are polyphasic sleepers. They nap for short periods throughout the day and night.

Toddlers are sort of in limboland between polyphasic and monophasic sleepers. They still benefit from naps. Truth be told, adults do too. Many high achieving people—including Napoleon, Thomas Edison, Albert Einstein, Winston Churchill, John F. Kennedy, Ronald Reagan, and George W. Bush—are known to have taken afternoon naps.

Many toddlers begin to fight their naps, however. We urge you to try to transition your little one to a period of "quiet time" in its place.

Think this through ahead of time and set firm, clear rules. Perhaps your toddler doesn't have to sleep, but he can sit quietly in bed and read or color. This sets the stage and opportunity for a nap, should the sandman pay a visit.

### JUSTIFICATION FOR A CELEBRATION

If you're one of the rare moms who's able to ease her toddler's transition from a nap to an hour or two of quiet time, know that you're among the elite, and you deserve to do something special for yourself.

## Napping Locations

At some point, most moms realize almost *any* safe toddler nap location is a good nap location!

⌁

All of my sons napped until they were three years old. Even in preschool, they had a mandatory "cot time" when they'd have to lie down. At home, my kids simply dropped their naps when they didn't need them anymore. At some point, they just stopped being excessively fussy during the day without a nap.

> —*Kristy Magee, MD, a mom of 15-, 12-, and 8-year-old sons and a family physician at North Seminole Family Practice and Sports Medicine, in Sanford, FL*

⌁

At nighttime, my babies really wanted to sleep next to me. But for naps, they often managed to nap in their cribs.

Sometimes they napped strapped to my husband or me in the Baby Björn. What I found worked best was to put the baby in the carrier and walk on the treadmill. I had exercised a lot when I was pregnant, and I think that the noise of the machine, rhythmic bouncing, and sound of my heartbeat re-created the womb-like state. After a few minutes of that, my babies would crash and fall asleep.

> —*Deborah Gilboa, MD, a mom of 14-, 12-, 10-, and 8-year-old sons, a family physician with Squirrel Hill Health Center, in Pittsburgh, PA, and a parenting speaker whose advice is found at AskDoctorG.com*

⌁

Our boys were always in day care and then preschool. It didn't have much impact on their sleep, especially because they had naptime at their full-day preschool. We took their blankets and stuffed animals to day care for them. We later bought duplicates so we wouldn't have to worry about taking blankets and stuffed animals home with us every evening.

On my kids' days at home, such as holidays or weekends, we'd make sure they would have a consistent naptime. It's not always easy to keep the naptime exactly the same time as in day care, but we knew

**Read a Good Book**

Yes, *Goodnight Moon, Where the Wild Things Are,* and *The Cat in the Hat* are good reads, but there comes a time when you need a good, twisting plot and a complex protagonist. As your child moves from naptime to quiet time, encourage him to peruse his bookshelf of kiddie books on his own while you turn to something that's more on your reading level, whether you prefer literary fiction, a good mystery, or the latest celebrity memoir. If you're looking for some good titles, check out Goodreads at **GOODREADS.COM.** The site lists top books by genre, and it will give you book recommendations based on what you've already read and enjoyed.

they needed that time to rest. Even if we didn't put them down for a nap, eventually they would come to us and want to get in our laps to settle down for a nap.

—*Leena S. Dev, MD, a mom of teenage boys and a general pediatrician, in Maryland*

❧

My four-year-old son still naps once a day for about 90 minutes, including at preschool. At preschool, all the kids have their own little cots or mats. I bought my son a roll-away mat, decorated in his favorite cartoon characters. After lunch, the teachers lay out the mats, and the kids all lie down to rest and nap. At first, my son would just talk to the little boy next to him, but after a few days (the teachers tell me!), he got the hang of it and would close his eyes and actually nap!

On weekends, I attempt to replicate the process. After lunch, I take my son into the master bed (we still co-sleep), lay him down with his "snuggie" blanket, and remind him that after his nap we'll have fun! Usually, I lie down next to him to nap too. Parenting is more exhausting than anesthetizing patients!

—*Edna Ma, MD, a mom of a 4-year-old son and an 18-month-old daughter, an anesthesiologist, and the founder of BareEASE pre-waxing numbing kit, in Los Angeles, CA*

We didn't do day care and used a nanny instead so that my child could nap when he needed to as opposed to being on a state-mandated schedule.

My biggest beef with day care centers is that they force kids to drop naps way too soon and then force them onto a sleep schedule that is not suitable for that particular age group. I feel many kids who are in day care are overtired and sleep deprived.

I was fortunate to have a nanny for my child. But I encourage parents to at least have an at-home caregiver (family member, nanny share) for their children for at least the first year, if not the first two years, if possible. During the first year, kids should be taking five naps in the newborn period and three naps by the time they're a year old. Most day cares allow kids to take only one nap when they're a year old. That's a travesty, in my opinion. I would love to change day care sleep regulations. I understand that having a nanny is not an option financially for all parents, but if other sacrifices can be made so a nanny can be available, I feel that's the best option. Plus, while the baby is taking his five naps a day, the nanny can make dinner for the family and clean the house. It's a win-win for the entire family, especially if there are two working parents with several kids. If day care is the only option, discuss with the facility beforehand that you want your child to get as much sleep as possible, even if that means he has to sleep in an infant room.

—*Nilong Parikh Vyas, MD, MPH, a mom of seven- and five-year-old sons and the founder and owner of Sleepless in NOLA sleep consulting, in New Orleans, LA*

❧

My boys sometimes napped in the car, but the challenge was that none of them transferred well *out* of the car! They would fall asleep, but as soon as I tried to get them out of the car, they'd wake up. We used to joke that they had speedometers.

One of my babies also presented another challenge: If I was standing up and rocking him, he'd sleep, but he'd wake if I tried to sit down. He apparently also had an *altimeter*!

—*Deborah Gilboa, MD*

Most new parents have had the experience of having a baby napping in the car. The problem then is needing to drive around and find a drive-thru Starbucks to pass the time so the baby gets a good nap once he has finally fallen asleep.

It's funny to hear so many other parents describe this same thing. It's just not something you ever think about having to do until you're at that point. I am looking forward to more of that soon with my new baby!

—*Sigrid Payne DaVeiga, MD, a mom of 10-year-old and 1-month-old sons and a 5-year-old daughter and a pediatric allergist with the Children's Hospital of Philadelphia, in Pennsylvania*

## BABY SLEEP PRO TIP
### Napping Areas for Toddlers and Preschoolers

If your child goes to preschool, ask about their nap policies, which should include the following.

Provide each child with a mat or cot in the classroom. Some state licensing boards require cots; other states allow toddlers and preschoolers to nap on mats.

Store cots or mats in a location away from walkways and without interfering with other learning areas in the room. Cover cots when not in use to reduce the spread of germs.

Create a system to assign children the same cot each day. Label cots with children's names, or number the cots and create a key so you know which cot belongs to which child.

Clean and sanitize cots before putting them away. Launder sheets daily. Stacking mats or cots with used sheets can promote the spread of germs.

Wash linens frequently. Send blankets, pillows, and stuffed animals home with families every week for washing.

Whether your toddler is at home or school, a quiet, calming environment will help promote rest. Dimming lights and playing white noise, CDs, or even an app, such as Relax Melodies, can help lull children of all ages to sleep.

**—Rebecca Kempton, MD**

## Resisting Napping

Don't panic if your toddler is resisting a nap! Some children go through periods during which they refuse to nap—even though they still need the rest. If you think this is the case, try tweaking your toddler's bedtime. Making bedtime a little earlier or later can sometimes help a child nap better during the day.

Our daughter was a great sleeper, but she dropped her naps much earlier than her peers. That was sad for me because her naptime gave me a chance to recharge. Plus, she was moody, and our evenings were harder for a few months. But after a while, she settled into her new routine.

—*Katja Rowell, MD, a mom of a 10-year-old daughter, a family practice physician, and the author of* Helping Your Child with Extreme Picky Eating and Love Me, Feed Me *at* TheFeedingDoctor.com, *in St. Paul, MN*

When my daughter was about 15 months old, she started resisting napping. Sometimes my husband or I would try driving her around the block at naptime to get her to sleep a bit, or we would time running our errands so that a nap might occur on the way home.

My son started resisting his nap when he was around two years old, but he would sometimes nap later in the day to make up for it. The challenge with this, though, was avoiding too late a nap, so that it didn't affect bedtime. On days when my son takes a later nap, it's often more difficult to get him to sleep at a reasonable time. But on

### Become a Master Napper

Taking restful naps takes skill and practice. You may not fall asleep during the first few tries, but lying down at the same time every day, setting your alarm for the same length of time for each nap, and trying not to stress about whether or not you sleep may help you get into a napping habit.

the other hand, when he skips his nap, it's sometimes *still* difficult to get him to sleep at night because he's then overtired.

—*Manpreet K. Gill, MD, a mom of a five-year-old daughter and a three-year-old son and a family practice physician with North Seminole Family Practice, in Sanford, FL*

I'm in the midst of this transition period now with my toddler! He's four years old, and occasionally he'll resist napping. At preschool, the children his age are required to lie down and rest for 90 minutes, even if they don't actually sleep.

I maintain the same schedule at home on weekends, even though this sometimes disrupts lessons or parties. On weekends, when it's naptime, I put my son in his bed, and I close the door. I tell him that I'll be back after he wakes and then we will do something fun. But I remind him that we can't do anything fun if he's too tired. Usually this short conversation is enough motivation for him to get to sleep.

I make the bedroom environment cozy for my son by giving him his favorite pillow, "snuggie," and cuddle toy. I darken the room, hug and kiss him, and reassure him that I'll be back. I also have him tell me, "Yes, Mommy, I will take a nap. I will close my eyes and have a nice nap."

—*Edna Ma, MD*

My twins haven't given up their nap yet. If they don't nap, they're very tired and cranky in the evening. Of course, because they still nap, their bedtime is a little after 8:30 pm.

Next year, when they start transitional kindergarten, they'll have to give up naps. We're planning on giving up naps and moving up their bedtime.

—*Sonal R. Patel, MD, a mom of four-year-old twin daughters and a physician who specializes in pediatric/adult allergy and immunology with Adventist Health Physicians Network, in Los Angeles, CA*

## BABY SLEEP PRO TIP: Transition to No Naps

According to sleep expert Marc Weissbluth, MD, 91 percent of three year olds still nap. Most kids still need a nap at age three and even age four. Just because your child is fighting a nap doesn't mean he doesn't need a nap anymore.

Here are some signs that your child may be ready to drop the nap.

• Consistently playing through nap time and not acting tired. In other words, there are no late afternoon meltdowns after skipping a nap.

• Taking too long to fall asleep at bedtime. If it takes your child longer than an hour to fall asleep at bedtime, it may be time to shorten the nap or drop it entirely.

• Your child doesn't act tired after missing a nap. If skipping a nap leads to afternoon tantrums, your child probably isn't ready. But if your little one is happy the rest of the day until bedtime, she may be ready.

**Tips for a successful transition to no naps.**

• Put together a quiet time basket, which you only bring out during rest time. Fill it with things your child can play with independently, such as puzzles, books, coloring books, and crayons.

• At rest time, bring out the basket and tell her she has the choice to sleep or not to sleep, but because it's rest time, she has to stay in her room and either nap or play on her own with quiet time activities.

• Set a tot clock or timer to signal the end of quiet time. (See "Teach Me Time; Talking Alarm Clock and Night Light on page 200.) An hour to an hour and a half is long enough. Tell her that when the tot clock changes colors or the alarm sounds, she can come out of her room.

• If she comes out before quiet time is over, remind her it's quiet time and take her back to her room silently.

Be consistent about the time and your response so your child understands the rules.

—*Rebecca Kempton, MD*

# Chapter 20

## Focusing on Safe Sleeping

In an episode of *Sex and the City*, Miranda and her boyfriend diligently put protectors in the electrical outlets all over their baby's nursery—while the baby sleeps under a blanket, in a crib wrapped in bumpers, with a mobile overhead—examples of what not to do!

When your toddler transitions out of the crib to a bed, you really have to ramp up your babyproofing. After all, now your toddler can get out of bed completely unattended! Here are a few important things to babyproof in the nursery.

- Put protectors in the electrical outlets.
- Secure all furniture to the wall and/or floor so it can't topple over.
- Protect sharp furniture edges with padding.
- Tie up/secure window coverings, such as blind cords and curtains.
- Move furniture away from windows.
- Never depend on a window screen to keep a toddler from falling out. Install window stops, which prevent windows from opening more than a few inches.

### JUSTIFICATION FOR A CELEBRATION
Your toddler stayed in her own room? All night! Hallelujah!

> **Out of this nettle, danger, we pluck this flower, safety.**
> **—*William Shakespeare***

## Babyproofing the Nursery

At some point around the time you move your toddler out of her crib, it will hit you, *Uh oh. Now what?* One of the most challenging parts of parenting—really of life—is letting go. Your toddler's new freedom means you have to let go of some mom control. Just imagine, someday you'll hand her the keys to your car!

❦

When my twins were sleeping in a bed and could now get up at night, my husband and I took turns wearing earplugs. We needed to balance our need for sleep with the need to be able to hear them in case of an emergency.

To keep my twins in their room, I put safety door locks on the inside doorknobs so that they couldn't get out of the room at night. If there's an emergency, it's important to know where your children are.

> —*Sonal R. Patel, MD, a mom of four-year-old twin daughters and a physician who specializes in pediatric/adult allergy and immunology with Adventist Health Physicians Network, in Los Angeles, CA*

### Mommy MD Guides-Recommended Product
#### Safety Bedrail by Summer Infant

If you're moving your child into a twin or larger-size bed, you can help her sleep peacefully and safely with a bed rail. You won't lose sleep worrying about whether or not she'll fall out of bed in her sleep. This bedrail fits twin to queen-size mattresses and platform beds. It even folds down for easy access for nighttime tuck-ins, hugs, and bedtime stories.

The panel is 42½ inches long and 21 inches high. It costs $29.99. You can buy it at stores nationwide and at **SummerInfant .com**.

Of course, we babyproofed the nursery—no knives or poisons! But Americans too often design stuff to protect our children to such a degree that no one learns or explores. Our kids are placed in overprotective shells. It's no wonder teens can't handle basic situations. Why are we surprised?

I focused on babyproofing those things that if you have one error, a child could be dead. For example, I covered electrical outlets. But, on the other hand, I allowed my little crawlers to explore and crawl under beds. If you crawl under, get stuck, and have to be rescued, that's a great teaching moment!

I allowed my toddlers to explore certain cabinets, but I trained them with "Uh, oh...we go here," and I pointed to the correct one.

Tiny items are never to be left out. And warm humidifiers must be out of reach and not in the same room as a toddler because of the risk of burns.

—*Hana R. Solomon, MD, a mom of four grown biological children, two grown "spiritually adopted" children, a grandmom of eight, a pediatrician, the president of BeWell Health, LLC, the inventor of Dr. Hana's Nasopure nose wash for children, and the author of* Clearing the Air One Nose at a Time: Caring for Your Personal Filter, *in Columbia, MO*

## Mommy MD Guides-Recommended Product
### Skip Hop Zoojamas Little Kid Pajamas

If you're looking for a cute and comfortable pair of pajamas for your toddler, check out Skip Hop's Zoojamas. They're 100 percent cotton and scratch-free, and the pajama tops are double lined. You can get them in owl, monkey, bumblebee, butterfly, and dog designs.

One pair of pajamas costs $25 and can be bought from Skip Hop's website here: **SKIPHOP.COM.**

## Choosing Safe Sleepwear

Many kids' pajamas sold in the United States contain chemicals to make theme flame-retardant. But are they safe?

A study published in the August 2014 issue of the journal *Environmental Health Perspectives* suggests maybe not. The researchers studied 389 pregnant women to ascertain the effects of the chemicals polybrominated diphenyl ethers (PBDEs), which are the flame retardants added to furniture, carpet padding, electronic devices, other consumer products—and yes children's pjs. The scientists discovered that higher levels of PBDEs were associated with lower IQ and higher hyperactivity scores in children.

Previous studies found that Americans have about 10 times higher levels of PBDEs in their bodies than do Europeans and Asians. That's likely because of previous United States' regulations that required flame retardants be added to products to prevent burn injuries and property damage.

Given the choice between flame-retardant sleepwear and tight-fitting sleepwear, the tight-fitting ones might well be the safer choice.

～

I always dressed my toddlers in 100 percent cotton pajamas with no chemicals. I felt—and still feel—that our kids are being exposed to too many chemicals all at once in their young years. The chemical load accumulates, and we don't know how this will affect our next generation. I err on the side of caution. Their pjs were also always well washed.
—*Hana R. Solomon, MD*

～

Our baby is 16 months old now, and at night we dress her in comfortable leggings, a long-sleeved shirt, and a fleece vest for sleep. This is our solution to keep her warm at night while balancing the SIDS-prevention guidelines of minimal bedding and keeping the ambient temperature comfortable for everyone else in the house.

The fleece vest is to keep my baby's core warm. As an anesthesiologist, I'm always concerned about maintaining core temperature! That's the most critical body part to keep warm.

Because our baby has minimal bedding, she doesn't have a blanket that could warm her. This way, we can sleep worry-free knowing that she has a safe sleep environment.

—*Edna Ma, MD, a mom of a 4-year-old son and an 18-month-old daughter, an anesthesiologist, and the founder of BareEASE pre-waxing numbing kit, in Los Angeles, CA*

## Mommy MD Guides–Recommended Product
### Teacher Created Resources Sand Timer

A sand timer is the perfect gadget to use to help your toddler keep track of periods of time. You can use sand timers to time lots of events, such as tooth brushing, eating, cleaning, and cuddling.

For instance, you might use the timer during cuddle time so your toddler knows how long you plan on staying and cuddling with him before you leave the room. Inform him that he can flip the timer, but when all the sand is gone, it's time to rest, relax, and go to sleep. If you have a 10-minute timer, simply flip it once to time for 20 minutes, such as 10 minutes for Mom and 10 minutes for Dad to cuddle. Before naps, I would stick to only 10 minutes of cuddle time.

Remind your child that once the sand is gone, there's no more flipping it. Even if your toddler asks, try not to give in. Warn him that it will only be flipped once (or twice), depending on how long you decide it will be and that is it. Stick to what you say. If he persists say, "I know you want it to go longer. I do too, but the sand is all gone." You could also use a kitchen timer or a timer on your phone.

—Nilong Parikh Vyas, MD, MPH, a mom of seven-
and five-year-old sons and the founder and owner of
Sleepless in NOLA sleep consulting, in New Orleans, LA

For an inexpensive, effective sand timer, you can't beat the Teacher Created Resources timers, a company that makes products by teachers for parents. They come in bright colors and a variety of time lengths. You can buy them on Amazon.com for around $10. For more information, visit **TEACHERCREATED.COM**.

# Chapter 21
## Balancing Screen Time and Sleep

How many times have you fallen asleep with the lights or television on, or even stayed up late to use your computer right before going to bed?

A key factor in regulating sleep and your biological clock is exposure to light or to darkness. That's why falling asleep with lights on may not be the best thing for a good night's sleep.

Exposure to light stimulates a nerve pathway from your eyes to the parts of your brain that control hormones, body temperature, and other functions that play a role in making you feel sleepy or wide-awake.

Too much light right before bedtime may prevent you from getting a good night's sleep. In fact, one study recently found that exposure to unnatural light cycles could have real consequences for your health, including increased risk for depression. Regulating exposure to light is an effective way to maintain natural circadian rhythms.

### JUSTIFICATION FOR A CELEBRATION
Your favorite TV show is on, and your kids are all asleep in time for you to watch it!

> **I love ghost stories but I can't really watch them, especially not by myself becasue then I can't sleep.**
>
> —*Laurie Holden, actress*

## Limiting Screen Time

According to the American Academy of Pediatrics (AAP), "Today's children are spending an average of seven hours a day on entertainment media, including televisions, computers, phones, and other electronic devices." That's practically a full-time job!

The AAP warns that, "Studies have shown that excessive media use can lead to attention problems, school difficulties, sleep and eating disorders, and obesity. In addition, the Internet and cell phones can provide platforms for illicit and risky behaviors."

The recommended screen time for toddlers through teens is less than two hours a day.

〜∽

The only TV my older son watched was *Your Baby Can Read*. We don't watch TV in our home in general. We'd have to purposefully turn it on in order to llmit it.

When my boys were toddlers, I let them play with my iPhone. They liked to play games that taught numbers, shapes, etc. It wasn't a struggle to get them to give it up. I simply said, "That's Mommy's phone. Now give it back."

—*Sharon Boyce, MD, a mom of seven- and five-year-old sons and a family physician with Oaklawn Medical Group, in Albion and Bellevue, MI*

〜∽

We have always limited screen time in our house, and we especially try to avoid excess stimulation in the couple of hours before bed. We try to stick to two hours a day maximum screen/electronics exposure, and we avoid screen time in the one to two hours before anticipated bedtime. This doesn't always work, but consistency does help.

—*Manpreet K. Gill, MD, a mom of a five-year-old daughter and a three-year-old son and a family practice physician with North Seminole Family Practice, in Sanford, FL*

〜∽

My husband and I don't watch a lot of TV, and our kids don't either. We did put on a *Baby Mozart* DVD sometimes, though! My babies would get so engaged in the program that I could get a considerable amount of housework done while it played. Or I could take a nap next to my baby on the floor if needed.

—*Marcela Dominguez, MD, a mom of a 13-year-old daughter and an 11-year-old son who has a private family medicine and wellness practice in Southern California, whose concierge medicine services are provided by Signature MD*

We never really watch TV in the evenings. I try not to overstimulate my kids after dinner. We play a little, read, and then do bath, books, bed. We never created an opportunity where we'd sit on the couch and watch TV.

—*Kristy Magee, MD, a mom of 15-, 12-, and 8-year-old sons and a family physician at North Seminole Family Practice and Sports Medicine, in Sanford, FL*

When my kids were little, I permitted them to watch an hour of cartoons before bath time. I made sure that screen time ended two to three hours before their bedtime to minimize the photo stimulation to the brain.

Now that my kids are older, they don't have any screen time

### Put Electronics to Bed

What better way to decompress than to turn away from the endless string of emails and barrage of status updates you get every day? There's also another very good reason to turn off your electronics—including your computer, phone, and tablets—about two to three hours before bed: Studies have linked nighttime exposure to the blue light emitted by the screens with suppression of melatonin, which is the hormone that helps you to go to sleep.

Set a bedtime for your electronic devices. Use that time at night to get the baby to bed and focus on your own self-care, such as washing your face or taking a bath, and then read a book before turning in.

The type of light that emanates from the screens of electronic devices is activating to the brain and can make it difficult to fall asleep.

Avoiding the use of electronic devices before bed will make it easier to fall asleep or return to sleep if you've awoken in the middle of the night.

during the week—unless they need to use a computer for homework, of course. I felt bad for my kindergartner last year because she didn't have much homework. But if you turn the TV on for one kid, you can't really prevent the others from watching it.

None of my kids have any screens in their bedrooms—nor will they ever!

—*Aline T. Tanios Keyrouz, MD, a mom of 13- and 7-year-old and 9-month-old daughters and an 11-year-son and an assistant professor of pediatrics at St. Louis University, in Missouri*

One thing we didn't do was let our kids fall asleep with electronics on. I know parents who do that, and I had friends growing up who needed the TV on to fall asleep. We didn't want anything to become a crutch our kids needed to sleep.

We played an international music CD to help our daughter sleep. After a while, she became so accustomed to falling asleep to it that she had difficulty falling back to sleep in the night without it and asked us to turn it back on. After that, we began weaning her off of the music. We weaned my son off of his classical "sleep music" when his CD player broke.

Today, my daughter has a phone, but she's not allowed to have it in her room at night. In fact, we have a "no electronics in bedrooms" rule.

—*Lauren Hyman, MD, a mom of a 13-year-old daughter and an 11-year-old son and an ob-gyn at West Hills Hospital and Medical Center, in California*

> **Think in the morning. Act in the noon.**
> **Eat in the evening. Sleep in the night.**
>
> —*William Blake, poet and painter*

We live in a very overstimulated society. Our brains really do need downtime, and we don't need nearly as much stimulation as we get these days. Babies especially need time when their brains can wander. Babies are designed to be attached to mom's hip or shoulder, looking at the world, napping when they're tired, and not doing much else. I carried my kids a lot when I could rather than putting them in a stroller. Skin-to-skin or body-to-body contact is so important. We secrete oxytocin, the cuddle hormone, when we touch one another, and this hormone creates a sense of well-being for both mom and baby.

>   —*Eva Ritvo, MD, a mom of two grown daughters, a psychiatrist,*
>   *and a coauthor of* The Beauty Prescription, *in Miami Beach, FL*

We didn't start screen time for our kids until they were older than two. Because we had caregivers in our home while we worked, we told them what we expected and they complied. My younger son started watching TV a little earlier because he had an older brother. But he was not truly interested in sitting and watching an entire TV show until he was closer to three or four years of age.

We still restrict TV time to only weekends, and our children get to watch one show each. They get to watch a movie once a month when we go on date nights. They get the iPad only if they're dressed and ready in the morning for school before we have to leave. And they can earn iPad time for doing what needs to be done to get ready for bed.

>   —*Nilong Parikh Vyas, MD, MPH, a mom of seven- and five-*
>   *year-old sons and the founder and owner of Sleepless in NOLA*
>   *sleep consulting, in New Orleans, LA*

I never limited screen time. The only screen that existed when my kids were little was the TV screen.

Today, my grandkids play with all kinds of screens. I think my daughter limits screen time by offering lots of activities to choose from so that screen time is not the only entertainment around.

—*Kathryn Boling, MD, a mom of two grown daughters, a grandmom of two, and a family medicine physician with Mercy Medical Center, in Baltimore, MD*

## Screen Time Impacting Sleep

Any mom who's fallen asleep watching *Scandal* can attest that TV-induced sleep is not *quality* sleep. Clearly, the screen impacts sleep—and not in a good way.

❦

Adults should stop exposure to the blue light that's emitted from TVs and other screens several hours before bedtime. This is the same for babies. In fact, babies are even more sensitive to blue light than adults. They need to be away from blue light so their brains know it's time for sleep. I'm not a fan of television, and my girls grew up in the pre-iPhone and iPad era, so it wasn't much of an issue for us. Things are much more complicated now.

—*Eva Ritvo, MD*

❦

When our kids were babies, we often put them to sleep in a smaller, mobile crib we kept in our living room with us while we watched TV. We noticed that the light coming off of the TV was enough to wake them up. Even if they weren't facing the TV, the light bouncing off the wall affected them!

After we discovered that, we put our babies in their dark bedrooms to sleep instead.

—*Marcela Dominguez, MD*

❦

I don't allow *any* screen time 30 minutes before napping and 60 minutes before bedtime. I think it's crucial to restrict screen time to get adequate sleep, for children, and for adults as well. If you're sitting in your bed and feeling sleepy but then you get on your phone or tablet, guaranteed, you'll be stimulated awake.

The blue light from the screens can stimulate your retinas and make your body think it's time to be awake. You'll go into an alert cycle (get a second wind), and it'll be another 90 minutes, or longer, before you can fall asleep again. It works the same for kids. Some parents like to read to kids with an electronic device before bed, but it's best to stick to paper books for that purpose.

—*Nilong Parikh Vyas, MD, MPH*

❧

My son doesn't have much interest in TV. He does play on an iPad for 30 minutes a day during the week if he desires, maybe an hour on weekends. I am not sure if it affects his sleep.

—*Larissa Guerrero, MD, a mom of a three-year-old son and family practice physician with Healthrow Ob/Gyn, in Orlando, FL*

## Mommy MD Guides–Recommended Product
### Teach Me Time: Talking Alarm Clock and Night Light

This alarm clock turns green when it's time to get up for the morning. If your child gets up before then, you can ask, "Is the nightlight green? If not, you need to go back and lie down. You can get up when the nightlight is green."

Remember to plug it in out of your child's reach or put in batteries so he doesn't mess with the settings but can still see the time.

—Nilong Parikh Vyas, MD, MPH, a mom of seven- and five-year-old sons and the founder and owner of Sleepless in NOLA sleep consulting, in New Orleans, LA

When your child is older, he can play an interactive time-teaching game with five adjustable skill levels. Later, the clock can be used as a fully-functioning alarm clock with a snooze button.

You can buy a Teach Me Time Alarm Clock on **AMAZON.COM** for around $38.

## BABY SLEEP PRO TIP: Manage Screen Time

Recent research has confirmed the detrimental effects of screen time on sleep in kids, but it probably won't make any parent take down a flat screen or delete their apps on mobile devices.

An educational TV show, an iPad app, or a computer program in small doses and at the right time is fun, educational, and stimulating. Here are three tips that allow your family to have their screen time and sleep too.

**Watch TV outside the bedroom.** Eliminate TVs in children's bedrooms. In a study published by the journal *Pediatrics*, kids with TVs in their bedrooms lost the most sleep. After all, it is cozy to cuddle up in bed, turn on some toons, and forget how much time passes. But parents can manage their children's TV viewing more easily if the TV is in the main living area of the house, rather than in their children's bedrooms. Also, TVs in children's bedrooms are linked to childhood obesity.

**Employ the two-hour rule.** Any screen, including computers, iPads, TVs, and video games, should be turned off at least two hours prior to bedtime. Because the blue light from screens mimics sunlight, it disrupts the internal biological clock and inhibits production of melatonin, our body's sleep-inducing hormone. With this two-hour rule, the bodies' melatonin secretion occurs naturally.

**Monitor the media diet.** The American Academy of Pediatrics recommends no screen time for children under age two and only one to two hours a day for children and teens—and that content should be high quality. Fortunately, there are thousands of educational apps that are also fun for kids, which makes it easier for you to turn off Sponge Bob and try Snail Bob. The best way to monitor screen time is to watch together: Find an educational show or app you both enjoy.

—*Rebecca Kempton, MD*

# Chapter 22
## Potty Training and Sleep

The American Academy of Pediatrics recommends beginning potty training when a child is around 18 to 24 months old. That's because bladder and bowel control take hold by 18 months.

Potty training is rarely a quick process, however. It involves changing both your toddler's physical process and his behavior. It's interesting to note that girls generally potty train three months earlier than boys. Most kids are potty trained by age three. Of course, this is all for the more simple day time!

Nighttime potty training is totally different. Almost a quarter of three year olds wet the bed and 10 percent of seven year olds do. This is one of those areas where a tincture of time and a pound of patience really pay off. Be patient. Be gentle. Be kind.

### JUSTIFICATION FOR A CELEBRATION
Your toddler stayed dry all night! Hurrah!

> **You can lead a toddler to the potty, but you can't make him pee.**
> —*Anonymous*

## Nighttime Potty Training

You might finally feel like your toddler is sleeping well. Then it's time for potty training, which introduces a host of new sleep challenges.

❧

My oldest daughter literally potty trained herself at about 18 months. She asked for the potty chair and started telling me that she had to make pee or poop. She had a couple of accidents, but it was very easy with her.

—*Kathryn Boling, MD, a mom of two grown daughters, a grandmom of two, and a family medicine physician with Mercy Medical Center, in Baltimore, MD*

❧

I didn't potty train my boys for nighttime until they were three or four years old. They sometimes did get up to go to the bathroom. A parent can tell when it's real or when it's an excuse. I think it's fine either way. I just always made sure the bathroom trips were super boring. I didn't turn on any lights. I didn't talk, smile, or engage them in any way. And I certainly didn't redo the bedtime routine. I helped them go to the bathroom, and then I returned them to bed.

—*Deborah Gilboa, MD, a mom of 14-, 12-, 10-, and 8-year-old sons, a family physician with Squirrel Hill Health Center, in Pittsburgh, PA, and a parenting speaker whose advice is found at AskDoctorG.com*

❧

I had it in my head that when my daughter was two years old, I wasn't going to need to buy diapers anymore. I took the potty chair and my naked daughter out to the backyard. I thought, *Eventually, she will have to go!* She did not. After several hours of drinking water and trying, we went indoors, and immediately she went potty in her diaper.

Clearly she wasn't ready yet. I decided to take a more relaxed approach. One day, when my daughter was about 2½ years old, her preschool teacher called to say she went potty on the toilet.

Because my son was able to watch his sister use the bathroom, potty training was so easy with him it was a nonevent. Once both of

## When to Call Your Doctor
## Bedwetting

Most children can make it through the night without wetting the bed by the time they have reached their sixth birthday, but that's not a hard-and-fast rule. Some healthy children may experience occasional bedwetting until they're 10 years old.

However, if bedwetting is accompanied by a fever, stomach pain, or pain while urinating, it could be a sign that your child has a urinary tract infection and should see a doctor. Also, if your child has gone three months or longer without wetting the bed and suddenly begins to do it again, it could be a sign of stress that you may want to discuss with your doctor.

my children were potty trained, their routine included using the toilet after their bath and wearing a pull-up diaper for a few weeks. Once we saw their diapers were dry most mornings, we transitioned them to training underwear and then eventually to regular underwear.

We had very few bedwetting events. However, when it occurred, we usually would reduce the nighttime fluid intake, installed a nightlight to the bathroom, and gave simple reminders to use the toilet at night if needed.

—*Marcela Dominguez, MD, a mom of a 13-year-old daughter and an 11-year-old son who has a private family medicine and wellness practice in Southern California, whose concierge medicine services are provided by Signature MD*

My older son wasn't nighttime potty trained until closer to four years of age. At that point, I had a talk with him about diapers and how he felt about trying to go without them at night. He was interested in trying. We put underwear on him at night and then a pull-up on top so that if he wet himself, he would feel it, but I wouldn't have to change the sheets. (The pull-up would catch any urine.) We agreed that if he wet the sheets, he would have to help me change the sheets.

I was going into my son's room every night, sometimes a couple of times per night, to help change sheets if he wet through them. So then I put another mattress on the floor and set out a fresh pair of clothes. If he wet himself, he was to change his clothes on his own and sleep on the mattress on the floor as opposed to his bed. After two nights of him having to do things on his own, he stopped wetting the bed.

We also eliminated drinks one hour before bedtime. He would urinate before bed, and then we would get him up to pee before we went to sleep for the night.

My younger son, however, both daytime and nighttime potty trained pretty much on his own at 18 months. This tells you that every child is different and needs to be looked at individually and that no single rule applies to each kid. My older son was daytime potty trained at that time, so I am sure that was an incentive for my younger son, but my older son was in nighttime pulls-ups long after my younger son was out of them.

—*Nilong Parikh Vyas, MD, MPH, a mom of seven- and five-year-old sons and the founder and owner of Sleepless in NOLA sleep consulting, in New Orleans, LA*

## Bedwetting

Bedwetting is when a child pees in the night without realizing it. It's also sometimes called nocturnal enuresis. It's actually hereditary. If you or your child's dad wet the bed as a child, your child has a 25 percent chance of bedwetting. If both of you were bedwetters as children, your child's chances increase to about 65 percent. Scientists have discovered a gene for enuresis.

∽

My second daughter fought the potty training process when we started at three years of age. She had lots of accidents and nighttime bedwetting. We helped limit that by taking her to the bathroom right before bed and then getting her up to go again right before we went to sleep later in the evening. It did not disrupt her sleep at all because she was barely awake when we got her up.

—*Kathryn Boling, MD*

When my boys were potty training, if they had accidents at night, they had to get up and take a bath or quick shower. That annoyed them a lot, so they learned to not drink before bed and to go to the bathroom before sleep to try to prevent accidents.

—*Sharon Boyce, MD, a mom of seven- and five-year-old sons and a family physician with Oaklawn Medical Group, in Albion and Bellevue, MI*

We never really had any problems with bedwetting. We were very consistent about taking our toddlers to the bathroom on a regular basis, about every 60 to 90 minutes, so they understood pretty quickly that it was the expectation to go in the potty. We read a few potty books too.

Once the boys were asleep, we would go back in their room and take them to the bathroom before we ourselves went to bed. This helped a lot.

—*Leena S. Dev, MD, a mom of teenage boys and a general pediatrician, in Maryland*

## Mommy MD Guides-Recommended Product
### GoodNites Bedtime Pants

Tiny bladders can't always make it through the night, and a nighttime pull-up can help lower frustration for both you and your little one.

GoodNites Bedtime Pants have characters such as super heroes and princesses that will excite your child about the transition to dry nights. S/M fits children 38 to 65 pounds and L/XL fits kids 60 to 125 pounds.

GoodNites also offers real underwear for kids with disposable inserts that discreetly hold wetness, also in two sizes, S/M and L/XL.

GoodNites are available at large retailers, pharmacies, and online. A pack of 33 bedtime pants costs $18.99, and a pack of two Tru-Fit real underwear with five disposable inserts costs $13.99.

# Chapter 23
## Solving Toddlers' Sleep Challenges

As babies grow into toddlers, the challenges to their sleep aren't necessarily lessened—they're just different. Common things that derail toddlers' sleep include sibling challenges, vacations and visitors, allergies, and illnesses.

Fortunately, as your toddler grows, he's better able to communicate with you what's bothering him and maybe what's keeping him up at night. Unfortunately, his reasoning abilities aren't up to par yet, so understanding what the problem is might not mean you can fix it!

### JUSTIFICATION FOR A CELEBRATION
Any time dreams outnumber nightmares is a reason to be happy and feel great.

> **Laugh and the world laughs with you;
> snore, and you sleep alone!**
>
> —*Anthony Burgess, writer and composer*

## Waking at Night

When your newborn baby cries in the night, and you race in to whisk his little body out of bed to comfort him, there's joy in that. When your toddler cries in the night for no apparent reason, jerking you out of sweet slumber, it's not quite as joy-filled.

❧

My younger daughter woke up a lot at night, even as a toddler. She just never really took to the idea of sleeping for eight or nine hours. She would often wake up and ask for a drink. I tried not to stress out over it. I just gave her a drink of water. We do the best we can.

—*Eva Ritvo, MD, a mom of two grown daughters, a psychiatrist, and a coauthor of* The Beauty Prescription, *in Miami Beach, FL*

❧

By the time my kids reached the toddler stage, they slept through the night most of the time, and they didn't wake to eat or be changed. But that didn't mean *I* got to sleep through the night. There was still an infant who needed to be fed or be changed!

—*Susan Besser, MD, a mom of six grown children, a grandmom of five, and a family physician at River Family Physicians, in Easton, MD*

❧

I never allowed my newborn in bed with me. As my daughter got older, my husband and I still tried very hard not to make a habit of allowing our daughter to sleep in bed with us, particularly through the night. We definitely get a visitor from time to time, and we soothe her and snuggle her for a bit, but then we put her back to bed!

—*Lisa M. Campanella-Coppo, MD, a mom of a six-year-old daughter and an emergency department physician at Summit Medical Group, in Livingston, NJ*

❧

When we transitioned my boys to a bed, I talked about the big boy bed but tried not to draw too much attention to it because I didn't want them to think it was a license to hop out of bed and come into my room.

We never did co-sleeping or allowed our boys in our bed. If they show up in my room at night, I gently walk them back to bed.

—*Kristy Magee, MD, a mom of 15-, 12-, and 8-year-old sons and a family physician at North Seminole Family Practice and Sports Medicine, in Sanford, FL*

When my kids were toddlers, they would sometimes find their way into my bed at night. I would generally walk them back to their rooms.

But for a while, it just was becoming a huge control issue. Sleep was becoming a negative thing for them. I didn't want them sleeping in my bed, so I put an air mattress on the floor. I let them sleep there. The novelty of that wore off pretty quickly, and they went back to sleeping in their own beds.

—*Eva Mayer, MD, a mom of a 12-year-old daughter and an 11-year-old son, an associate professor of pediatrics at Temple University, and a pediatrician with St. Luke's Hospital Coopersburg Pediatrics, in Pennsylvania*

### Cope with Apnea

Snoring can be more than an aggravation. If you or your husband is snoring or gasping for air at night, it could be a sign of sleep apnea, which isn't something to ignore. Untreated sleep apnea increases the risk of many medical conditions, such as high blood pressure, obesity, diabetes, and heart arrhythmia. Sleep apnea can raise your risk of a heart attack, stroke, or heart failure.

Your first step should be to get yourself or your spouse diagnosed and treated. Then it may be time to make some lifestyle changes that can improve the way you sleep, such as getting on a weight loss program, starting an exercise routine, quitting smoking, avoiding alcohol, and stopping medications that could make apnea worse. When you settle down for the night, use a saline nasal spray or a decongestant to help you breathe better, and sleep on your side or stomach instead of on your back to try to get a better night's sleep.

My younger daughter flung herself out of the crib when she was 18 months old, so she had to sleep in a bed from that day forward for safety.

Once my daughter was sleeping in a bed, she tried to get out of her room at night. That caused some real sleep disruption for several weeks until she got used to sleeping in the bed. We put a device on her door so she could not get out of the room at night while we were sleeping, but she could still see out the door.

—*Kathryn Boling, MD, a mom of two grown daughters, a grandmom of two, and a family medicine physician with Mercy Medical Center, in Baltimore, MD*

When our boys were toddlers, they would sometimes get out of bed. I simply reminded them that they weren't allowed to do that. If there wasn't an actual problem, I told them to go back to bed, and they did.

If my boys pushed it, I'd say, "If you're not big enough to stay in your big boy bed, you need to go back to your crib!" Usually just saying that was enough to get them back to bed. They were like, "No thanks, I'm good." But a few of my boys did need to sleep in the crib for a night. Natural consequences are often very effective.

—*Deborah Gilboa, MD, a mom of 14-, 12-, 10-, and 8-year-old sons, a family physician with Squirrel Hill Health Center, in Pittsburgh, PA, and a parenting speaker whose advice is found at AskDoctorG.com*

My daughter often woke up early. In fact, she still does at 10 years old! For a time when she was a preschooler, after she dropped her naps, she would fall asleep earlier in the evening and wake up at about 5:30 am. She was a pretty happy kiddo, so we put a digital photo frame with a timer near her bed. We filled it with fun photos, and we set the timer to go on at 6 am.

We explained to our daughter that when the photos came on, she could come out of her room. But if she woke up before the pictures came on, she needed to stay in her room and play or look at books. We were shocked at how well it worked. Sometimes she stayed in bed and just looked at the pictures for a while.

—*Katja Rowell, MD, a mom of a 10-year-old daughter, a family practice physician, and the author of* Helping Your Child with Extreme Picky Eating and Love Me, Feed Me *at TheFeedingDoctor.com, in St. Paul, MN*

⌒∽⌒

The first few nights after transitioning my kids to a toddler bed were always challenging. They're free! They think they can do whatever they want. I'd put them in bed and think they were asleep, but a few minutes later they were following me downstairs! "No, no," I'd say. "Go back to your bed!"

Those first few nights, I spent more time near their rooms so I could hear what was going on. I'd sit and read outside the room.

When they would come out, I'd say, "This is your big kid bed! I want you to stay in it." It would sometimes take some negotiating back and forth for a few days, but then they'd get it.

—*Aline T. Tanios Keyrouz, MD, a mom of 13- and 7-year-old and 9-month-old daughters and an 11-year-son and an assistant professor of pediatrics at St. Louis University, in Missouri*

⌒∽⌒

My children are very different from one another. My daughter hated being alone in her crib in her room. She simply hated that crib!

When my daughter was two years old, we moved the crib mattress to her bedroom floor. All of a sudden, she was perfectly fine with sleeping in her room! Knowing that she had her freedom meant she didn't need it anymore.

My son, on the other hand, loved his crib. When he was two years old, he started to climb out of the crib. So we had to move him out of it for his safety. But then he hated being in his room alone! We couldn't keep him in there! We put a baby gate in his doorway. He climbed over it. We put the gate up higher. He crawled under it. Finally we stacked two gates, one atop the other. He wailed and wailed to be let out. Fortunately, this lasted only a few really sad days, and then he was okay.

—*Lauren Hyman, MD, a mom of a 13-year-old daughter and an 11-year-old son and an ob-gyn at West Hills Hospital and Medical Center, in California*

The most interesting sleep challenge we had happened after we transitioned our twins to toddler beds. Our son wouldn't sleep in his bed! He became convinced that monsters lived in the bed.

Our son had a large—four-foot-tall!—stuffed bear that was sewn for him by his aunt. He thought the bear would protect him from the monsters, so he slept on the bear on the floor. We tried to put the bear in the bed, but it would always end up on the floor with our son on top of it. This went on for years—from when our son was 2½ until he was 5 years old.

At first, we tried to devise all kinds of tricks and enticements to get him back to bed. But then we decided it really didn't matter. He slept when he was supposed to. People in many cultures sleep on floors. We take the kids camping, so they all have had the experience of sleeping on the ground.

The only issue was that our son was still potty training when it all started. We made a makeshift "nest" for him with a waterproof sheet and a regular sheet and a blanket all tucked up on this ridiculous stuffed bear.

When his grandparents visited, they tried to convince him to sleep in his bed. He would tell them he fell out of bed during the night, landing on his bear. They made a big deal out of the whole thing. The truth was, it really wasn't worth arguing over. I think when we tried insisting he sleep in his bed, we were being too rigid.

Finally after three years, our son just decided one day that he was a big boy and got into bed.

—*Rebecca Jeanmonod, MD, a mom of 12- and 8-year-old daughters and 11- and 8-year-old sons and a professor of emergency medicine and the associate residency program director for the emergency medicine residency at St. Luke's University Health Network, in Bethlehem, PA*

## Solving Sibling Challenges

The good thing about a sibling is he's a friend who never has to go home. The bad thing about a sibling is he's a friend who never goes home. Siblings can solve some sleep challenges, but they probably create more sleep challenges.

My boys have always doubled up in rooms. They are so used to this that for my youngest especially, if he ever had to sleep alone, I could tell he was wondering, *It's so quiet! I don't understand what's happening!*
　　—*Deborah Gilboa, MD*

Both our boys had separate rooms. This gave each of them some space of their own for separate play activities. Inevitably, they would end up in the big brother's room to play because it had all the cool building toys and books! But they slept apart.
　　—*Leena S. Dev, MD, a mom of teenage boys and a general pediatrician, in Maryland*

I have a new baby and older kids. This presents a challenge at naptime and bedtime. We live in a two-story house. When my baby came home from the hospital, I established a rule that when she's upstairs sleeping, no one else is allowed up there, unless they are doing a practically silent activity, such as reading or playing electronics—with the sound off.
　　—*Aline T. Tanios Keyrouz, MD*

My son had always slept better than his older sister. But when he was around 15 months old, he started to have trouble getting settled to sleep. I think it was because he realized that his sister was still awake after his bedtime, so he started resisting sleep too.

To help my son to settle down, we try to lower the lights, and avoid TV and other noise. We read books to try to get both kids to wind down to sleep at the same time. In our house, this is at around 8:30 pm.
　　—*Manpreet K. Gill, MD, a mom of a five-year-old daughter and a three-year-old son and a family practice physician with North Seminole Family Practice, in Sanford, FL*

When our baby arrived, we were forced to rethink our sleeping arrangement. Our sleeping arrangement is still constantly in flux! When our baby was still a newborn, I slept in the room with her so I could more easily nurse her at night and not disrupt her older brother. During this phase, her older brother slept with my husband.

As our baby grew, she no longer needed to be fed at night. We transitioned her into a crib, which is in our walk-in closet, for maximum soundproofing! I resumed sleeping next to my son. My husband sleeps on the floor next to the walk-in closet. He's a heavy sleeper, but he'll wake up when she cries and tend to her. He has the incredible capacity to function normally the next day, with only minimal amounts of sleep! He's a super dad!

Really, there is no simple solution that will work for every family. Every family has to find what works for them. And thankfully, the children outgrow this phase!

—*Edna Ma, MD, a mom of a 4-year-old son and an 18-month-old daughter, an anesthesiologist, and the founder of BareEASE pre-waxing numbing kit, in Los Angeles, CA*

## Calming Nightmares and Fears

An international chocolate shortage. Starbucks bankruptcy. The return of bell bottoms. These are the stuff of mom nightmares. And of course, the serious ones we wouldn't even think of typing.

Toddlers are more likely to fear the dark. Monsters under the bed. While moms are often woken or kept awake by worries about what might happen, little ones' sleep is more likely disturbed by fears of what did happen, such as seeing a scary commercial or being frightened by a story. It's an ironic fact of life that most nightmares happen in the second half of the night—right about when you're cruising into deep, good sleep.

~~

My boys have had the occasional nightmare. I would go to their rooms to soothe them, or they'd come to me. After they calmed down, I made sure to get them back to bed.

—*Deborah Gilboa, MD*

~~

On occasion for the particularly scary thunderstorm or disruptive life event, we've had a nighttime visitor. Our daughter will creep into bed with us. We always return her to her bed as soon as the storm has passed and she has calmed down. We don't let her sleep the entire night in bed with us regularly; however, there have been exceptions.

We lived at the Jersey Shore through Hurricane Irene and Hurricane Sandy. I was locked into the emergency department for two days for Hurricane Irene, and my husband tells me that he and my daughter slept together partly for comfort and partly because he didn't want to be in a separate room from her if something should have happened during the storm.

During Hurricane Sandy, we evacuated to my mother's home in North Jersey, and we all slept in the same bed. My daughter wouldn't have slept at all if we hadn't, and, to be honest, I think we all took comfort from each other that night. To this day, she will not sleep in that room at my mother's house because of how frightened she was the night of Hurricane Sandy.

—*Lisa M. Campanella-Coppo, MD*

## Easing Anxiety and Stress

No one is immune to stress and anxiety—not you, not your toddler, not the cat. Well, okay, probably not the cat.

By now you know yourself well enought to understand your anxiety triggers. But what might be anxiety-provoking for your child?

- Fear of separation
- Strangers
- Pets and other animals
- Darkness

Children who are anxious sometimes show it in unexpected ways. For example, anxious toddlers might be less apt to want to get dirty, they might be sensitive to sounds and sensations, and they might develop rituals to try to gain a sense of control.

Only my youngest child went to day care. On his first day, I walked him in, and he grabbed the hand of the day care worker and walked away to go help make coffee. He was thrilled, and he never looked back. I, on the other hand, went to my car and cried. This transition didn't affect his sleep, thankfully.

—*Susan Besser, MD*

Some nights are still tough getting my daughter to sleep, especially now that she's a toddler. Sometimes she wants to stay up late and spend time with us, especially when we've been at work all day. I try to stick with her bedtime routine, which is still bath, lotion, reading, bed. It's definitely easier to stick with bedtime routines on the days when I'm off from work. It's harder to stick to the schedule when I've been away from my daughter at work all day. But I try my best.

—*Sonali Ruder, DO, a mom of a three-year-old daughter, an emergency medicine physician, and the author of* Natural Baby Food, *in Fort Lauderdale, FL*

When my kids are struggling with anxiety and having a hard time sleeping, I do guided relaxation with them. I'm a big proponent of mindfulness. I help my kids to relax each part of their bodies, by

## When to Call Your Doctor: Stress

It can be difficult to know the difference between a typical toddler meltdown and behavioral issues that are the result of stress and anxiety, especially when your child is too young to vocalize how he's feeling. Kids also tend to show feelings such as anxiety and depression in different ways than adults do. Kids may be irritable, while adults may be sad. A good rule of thumb is to call the doctor when anxiety is persistent and affects your child on a daily basis because it may be a sign of an anxiety disorder.

focusing on each body part in turn, from head to feet, and then relaxing that body part. I also take them on a guided relaxation meditation "trip," by talking through walking on the beach or floating on a raft. I don't want them to fall asleep while I'm doing this, because I don't want it to become a sleep crutch. So I leave the room when I hear their breathing change and realize they're getting close to falling asleep.

—*Lauren Hyman, MD*

Generally, our daughter knows she has to sleep in her own room. However, there's one time that she's allowed to sleep the entire night with one of us. Because my husband and I are shift workers and emergency responders, sometimes we're called to work all night. This is very disruptive for our daughter, and she gets upset.

Consequently, my husband and I established a policy that our daughter is allowed to sleep in bed with the home parent when the other parent has to work an overnight shift. This is a boundary and a rule that our daughter knows she has to follow. It makes up for the fact that one of us is not home to kiss her good night.

I think it's important for children to know that when something truly scary is going on, you'll be there for them. However, I also think that boundaries and definitions of what requires a full-night snuggle are key.

—*Lisa M. Campanella-Coppo, MD*

Going on a date night can cause a major disruption to a child's sleep routine. You go out, the baby is with a sitter, you get home late, and if you haven't asked the sitter to put the baby to bed, the baby is still up, tired and cranky. And now your feeling of relaxation is gone as you have to jump right back into motherhood and do your whole bedtime routine with a cranky baby!

It's important to have time together as a couple. Parenthood is a long journey, and you have to balance the needs of your child with the needs of your relationship.

Instead, have the babysitter do the routine and put the baby to bed. Then you can come home and continue the date night.

—*Eva Ritvo, MD*

## Mommy MD Guides–Recommended Product
### Natural Calm

One of the best natural calming remedies I've found is Natural Calm. It's a tart-tasting liquid that offers 240 milligrams of magnesium per capful. Children younger than eight years old should take only half a capful with 120 milligrams of magnesium, per day. It helps soothe and relax the GI tract and promote normal elimination. You don't want to go overboard and give your kids too much magnesium, as it can cause diarrhea.

Many kids and adults suffer from symptoms that can result from a lack of magnesium, including stress, fatigue, inability to sleep, muscle tension, anxiousness, nervousness, irritability, and headaches.

—Rallie McAllister, MD, MPH, a mom of three
sons and a family physician, in Lexington, KY

You can buy Natural Calm online and in health food stores for $15 to $16. Visit **NATURALVITALITY.COM/NATURAL-CALM** for more information.

*The maker of Natural Calm is a paying partner of Momosa Publishing LLC. Regardless of whether we receive compensation from a vendor, we only recommend products or services that we have used personally and that we believe will be good for our readers.*

When my kids were babies, I kept their rooms quiet. When they were toddlers, though, they each went through a few years where they had trouble falling asleep.

I bought my daughter a Putumayo World Music CD. It's multicultural, and I liked that it exposed her to many different rhythms. I played it for her each night.

I chose a number of songs that I would listen to with her each night before saying good night. I allowed for one extra "please, Mommy, one more" song. This way, my daughter could expect when it was time for me to say good night and make my exit from her room. My biggest challenge was not falling asleep before that point myself!

All kids want Mama or Dada comforting them while they relax into sleep, reassuring them that the goblins aren't going to be there. But at some point, once they are in bed and feel they're safe, they need to go to sleep on their own. This prepares them to be good sleepers as adults.

—*Lauren Hyman, MD*

### When to Call Your Doctor: Headbanging

Some children use headbanging and rocking to help themselves to go to sleep. According to the Cleveland Clinic, it's not a cause for concern when otherwise healthy children do those behaviors only when falling asleep.

Headbanging becomes a concern when your child hits his head hard enough to cause injury or if the behavior interferes with his sleep. Call your doctor if headbanging leads to injury, if you're worried it may harm your child, or if your child shows signs of a sleep disorder such as sleep apnea by snoring. You may also want to call your doctor if you have concerns about his development, if headbanging is disrupting others in the home, or if you're concerned your child is having seizures.

**BABY SLEEP PRO TIP:** Toddlers and Time Changes

Here are two essential steps for a successful daylight savings time shift:

**Dark room.** Be prepared for the question children love to ask! "Why are we going to bed when the sun is still out?" Your toddler is right: Nights will be lighter, so ensure those windows are covered with room darkening shades or my favorite low tech solutions: black garbage bags, dark construction paper, or tinfoil and painter's tape!

**Get a tot clock.** Toddler clocks are always helpful reminders of the "appropriate" time to wake up for your tot, and to begin to teach him about a daily schedule. (See "Teach Me Time: Talking Alarm Clock and Night Light" on page 200.)

—Rebecca Kempton, MD

## Vacations and Visitors

A vacation to Disney World. A visit from Grandma. Better still: A trip to Disney World with Grandma! All of these things have the potential to disrupt your toddler's sleep—and yours! But we think you'll agree, they're worth it!

Changes such as visitors or vacations wrecked our babies' sleep. Luckily, our children thrive on routine, so when the visitors left or the vacations were over, we were able to get back to the same routine pretty quickly.

—*Shilpa Amin-Shah, MD, a mom of a 6-year-old son and 5-year-old and 18-month-old daughters and an emergency medicine physician at Emergency Medical Associates, in St. Johns, FL*

If there's a break in normalcy—such as going on a vacation—the key is to avoid deviating from the routine. Keep up bedtime habits as much as you can. Massage, songs, books, etc.—these things will help baby to feel normalized and comfortable.

*—Mona Gohara, MD, a mom of nine- and seven-year-old sons, a
dermatologist in private practice, in Danbury, CT, and an associate
clinical professor in the department of dermatology at Yale University*

We did some overseas travel, and the time difference is a challenge.
With time changes, there wasn't much to do other than be prepared
for our daughter to wake up and want to play in the middle of the
night. I was also adjusting, so we played in the early morning hours
and then tried to sleep again. Usually, in a few days she was back on
track. Unfortunately, it didn't go as easily for me!

*—Katja Rowell, MD*

To help my daughter sleep better at home, I played a Putumayo World
Music CD. So that we didn't have to haul a CD player on trips, we also
downloaded the music to my husband's phone. Listening to that music
was my daughter's cue that it was time to go to sleep.

Interestingly, my son didn't like the words to the songs on that
CD! So we played classical music to help him to fall asleep. Today, he
plays piano beautifully, and he gravitates toward classical music.
Maybe that's because he went to sleep listening to Mozart all of
those years!

*—Lauren Hyman, MD*

## When to Call Your Doctor: Tooth Grinding

If you can hear your child grinding his teeth (aka bruxism) while
sleeping or if your child has a sore jaw or tooth damage after waking and it's painful to chew, be sure to call the dentist. Your child's
dentist can look for signs of damage from bruxism and also see
what may be causing it, such as a misalignment of his teeth.

If the grinding is causing a sore jaw or damage, your dentist
may recommend that your child wear a night guard that's molded
to his teeth.

When you take kids on vacation and sleep in hotels or family members' houses, it's a challenge. When our daughter was a toddler, we would put her in the middle of one of the hotel's queen beds and surrounded her with pillows so she couldn't roll off of the bed. Our bed was right next to hers. She didn't move much during the night, but if she moved, I would glance over to make sure she was still in the middle of the bed.

I wouldn't advise doing this unless you're sleeping in the bed right next to your child and you're a light sleeper, as I am, to check periodically during the night.

When my son was born, we used a Pack 'n Play for his travel bed.
—*Marcela Dominguez, MD, a mom of a 13-year-old daughter and an 11-year-old son who has a private family medicine and wellness practice in Southern California, whose concierge medicine services are provided by Signature MD*

⁂

We always faced challenges during vacations, which often disrupted our schedule and routine. When we got home, we tried to get things back to our consistent routine as soon as possible. We've also used very low-dose melatonin if needed when traveling or when we needed to get back on track. We've tried the supplement in liquid form, available over the counter, 0.5 to 1 milligram only, and infrequently because I haven't seen any definitive studies regarding its effectiveness or the long-term consequences of chronic use. However, melatonin has been helpful for our kids on occasion. (Talk with your doctor before giving your child this or any supplements.)
—*Manpreet K. Gill, MD*

⁂

With my first baby, vacations killed our sleeping routine every single time. It always threw off his sleep, and it required some tough love to get him back on track. We had to employ tough love techniques when we got home.

My second baby was a better sleeper overall, and so vacations didn't mess his sleep up as much.

*—Heather Orman-Lubell, MD, a mom of 15- and 11-year-old sons and a pediatrician at St. Chris Care at Yardley Pediatrics, in Pennsylvania*

⤳

Vacations and having visitors certainly change *everyone's* sleep patterns—not just babies and toddlers. For us, spending time with family, having visitors, and going on vacations are all good things, and we would let the children decide when they were ready for bed. We knew when our kids needed to go to bed, especially when they have had enough excitement, so we could push it a bit and *encourage* them to go to bed, but in the end, we would go with their needs and let them sleep when they were ready.

I remember a time when we were at a museum in Edinburgh, Scotland. Our three-year-old son *needed* a nap. So we took turns going through this small, quaint museum. I sat in a chair with our toddler for an hour while my husband looked through the museum, and then we switched. I think the worst was when our toddler liked buses so much, so we took a ride in a double decker and he slept the whole time! Same thing when we took a ride on a steam engine just for him. In the end, kids will sleep when they want to, so we just went with the flow!

*—Leena S. Dev, MD*

⤳

My children didn't seem to have many issues with changing time zones or vacations. Bedtime was bedtime. However, we often settled for just being quiet in bed, reading, or listening to a story tape if the kids weren't quite ready to fall asleep.

*—Susan Besser, MD*

## Combating Allergies

Don't you love that allergy medicine commercial? "Six is greater than one." Really? No kidding! What were they thinking? What's no joke is that if your child has allergies, it absolutely can affect his sleep.

My daughter has allergies. We all have hypoallergenic pillows with no feathers. We let her sleep with one teddy bear, and I routinely wash and dry it.

My daughter is allergic to dust, so I have to be diligent about keeping the blankets and toys dust-free.

—*Lisa M. Campanella-Coppo, MD*

My youngest baby boy had asthma and allergies. I helped him wash his nose and taught him to do it himself. I understood that his allergy/asthma episodes always began with a snotty nose, so washing it made sense. Now we know that rinsing with the correct solution will remove about 80 percent of the allergens!

Allergic or asthmatic kids often have significant issues during sleep, and, in fact, this poor sleep can result in poor learning, poor appetite, and, on occasion, poor behavior.

Cleaning the child's personal filter (his or her nose) while cleaning the environment and the diet are my preferences over using antihistamines, decongestants, nasal steroids, immune modulators, antibiotics, etc. They have numerous side effects.

## When to Call Your Doctor: Allergies

Any adult with allergies knows that the sneezing, coughing, congestion, and other symptoms can keep you awake at night. It's no different for kids. If your child has allergy symptoms, take him to an allergist for treatment sooner rather than later to get control of the symptoms, recommends the American College of Allergy, Asthma, and Immunology. Symptoms to watch for include sneezing, coughing, runny nose, itchy eyes, upset stomach, asthma or problems breathing, or skin rashes or hives. Possible triggers could be tree or plant pollen, insect bites, pet hair, mold, dust mites, cigarette smoke, perfume, car exhaust, or foods such as milk, eggs, or peanuts.

Cleaning the environment and the diet and the nose helps reduce the toxic load on the body.

> *—Hana R. Solomon, MD, a mom of four grown biological children, two grown "spiritually adopted" children, a grandmom of eight, a pediatrician, the president of BeWell Health, LLC, the inventor of Dr. Hana's Nasopure nose wash for children, and the author of* Clearing the Air One Nose at a Time: Caring for Your Personal Filter, *in Columbia, MO*

## Mommy MD Guides-Recommended Product
### Nasopure

A simple patented system called Dr. Hana's Nasopure can help with allergies and nasal congestion. Developed by a pediatrician using a mother's wisdom, Hana R. Solomon, MD, Nasopure is a modern, comfortable, and easy nose wash that cleans away mucus as well as pollen, mold, dust, bacteria, and viruses. Dr. Hana has spent the past three decades teaching her two-year-old patients how to wash their noses and teaching the medical world about the benefits of nasal washing over medications, prescriptions, and surgery.

To use Nasopure, simply pour the Nasopure salt mixture (which is buffered and pharmaceutical grade to ensure an ideal mixture with no burning) in the patented Nasopure bottle, add water, and flush the solution into the nose. It will exit through the opposite nostril, leaving you clean and refreshed. It's so easy, even a two year old can do it.

Dr. Hana's Nasopure kit contains an eight-ounce bottle, 20 salt packets, and instructions, and it offers 100 percent satisfaction guaranteed.

It's made in the United States, and it's assembled by adults with disabilities.

For more information and to order, visit **NASOPURE.COM.**

## Mom or Dad Returning to Work

Family dynamics can be a beautiful—until an event like going back to work causes it all to fall into cacophony.

I have two daughters, and I had two very different experiences with their sleep. With my older daughter, I went back to work when she was around nine weeks old. Right around that time, she settled in and became a good sleeper.

My younger daughter, however, did not. I used to joke that she might learn to sleep through the night in college. When I was being really silly, I joked that her spouse might someday get her to sleep through the night.

—*Eva Ritvo, MD*

When I returned to work, we got a nanny. She is fantastic and was very skilled at getting our daughter to take a nap. She used bribery. If our daughter did "this," then she would get "that," and she never caved in to manipulation.

### ? When to Call Your Doctor: Apnea

Toddlers can have sleep apnea. Letting sleep apnea go untreated in your toddler can have serious consequences. Kids who snore loudly are more likely to have learning problems, according to a study in the *Journal of the American College of Chest Physicians*, the National Sleep Foundation says. Poor sleep is also associated with hyperactivity, attention problems, cardiovascular issues, and delayed growth.

Listen to your child sleep and call your doctor if he snores, you hear pauses in his breathing, your child gasps or snorts during sleep, or your child wakes from breathing problems during sleep. Children with sleep apnea may also sleep in unusual positions and sweat while sleeping.

Relatives, on the other hand, are impossible. Using them for child care is disruptive because they allow my daughter to run the roost. They skip her nap and let her stay up to all hours. I find that having a person with whom you have a professional relationship, whose job it is to implement your wishes and who is consistent, is really the best option.

—*Lisa M. Campanella-Coppo, MD*

Starting day care and preschool impacted our children mostly because they're late sleepers, and they had to be woken up for school most days. The key was just to make sure they were asleep by a certain time each night to allow them enough sleep.

—*Jennifer Bacani McKenney, MD, a mom of a five-year-old daughter and a three-year-old son and a family physician, in Fredonia, KS*

The key for my family is that we *didn't* tweak our routine. We kept it the same. As toddlers, our boys knew that after two stories, a prayer, and two songs, it was time for sleep. They might not *want* to go to sleep, but the expectation was that they would stay in bed.

—*Deborah Gilboa, MD*

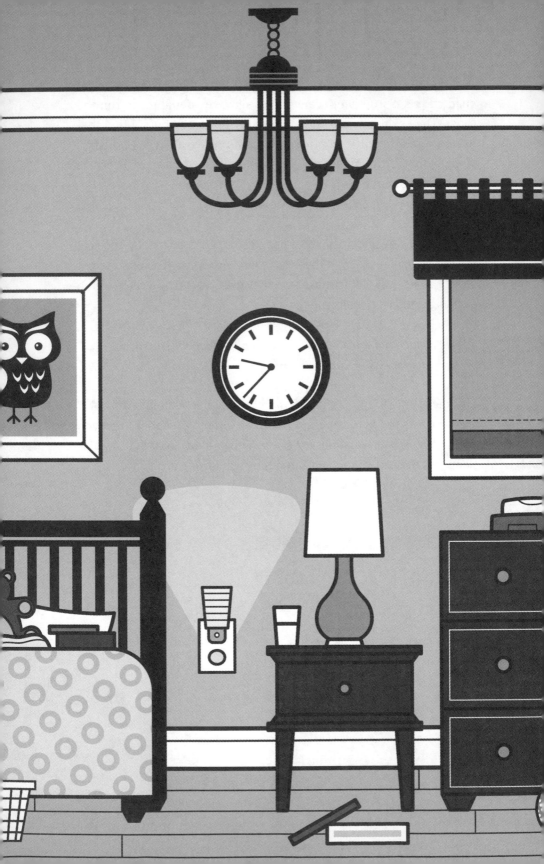

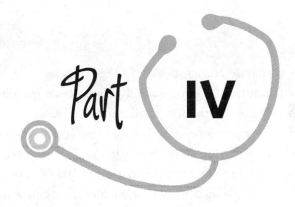

Part IV

# PRESCHOOL AND BEYOND

# Chapter 24
## Solving Preschoolers' Sleep Challenges

Just like kids change constantly, so do the challenges. What once seemed insurmountable, you probably have down pat now! And it's likely been replaced by new challenges.

Perhaps your preschooler is feeling stress and anxiety that are understandably affecting her sleep. Or maybe she started sleep walking or sleep talking. Even fun things like sleepovers can affect a kid's sleep, which of course means they can affect your sleep too.

At this stage of the game, you have weathered many storms and puzzled out many problems. No matter what challenges the sandman pitches to you, you can knock it out of the park!

### JUSTIFICATION FOR A CELEBRATION
One day, your little one will ask you to go to bed early for a good night's sleep! Celebrate by doing something fun or turning in early yourself!

> **Don't Quit!**
> When things go wrong, as they sometimes will,
> When the road you're trudging seems all uphill,
> When the funds are low and the debts are high,
> And you want to smile, but you have to sigh,
> When care is pressing you down a bit,
> Rest, if you must, but don't you quit.

## Easing Anxiety and Stress

Think back to your preschool days. Playing kickball in the park; catching fireflies after dark. Do you remember feeling anxious? We don't.

Perhaps it's just Mommy Memory, but life today feels a lot more stress-inducing than it was back then. In fact, children today do encounter more stressful situations at earlier ages than we did when we were kids.

Stress is often caused by conflict or imbalance. For example, it can be caused by a disconnect between the demands placed on us and our ability to meet them. Or it can be caused by the difference between what we think we should be doing versus what we're actually able to do.

Kids—even preschoolers—aren't immune to these feelings of conflict. Signs your child is stressed include anger, nervousness, stomachaches, and frequent illnesses. Stressed-out kids might cry easily or seem anxious or agitated.

Most adults don't know how to cope with stress—how could children possibly figure it out? But maybe as you learn to help your child, you can help yourself too. Get better sleep, eat more nutritious foods, spend quality time together, and express your thoughts and feelings. These are all great ways to try to stress less.

### How Much Sleep Does a Preschooler Need?

You might notice your growing preschooler sleeping a little less than she used to, and that's okay. Children who are three to five years old need about 10 to 13 hours of sleep each day, and they can get as little as 8 to 9 or as much as 14 hours. The time to be concerned and talk to your pediatrician is when your preschooler is consistently getting fewer than 8 hours or more than 14 hours of sleep each day.

When my son transitioned from the learning center to pre-K, he got less time to nap. This affected his sleep in that he was sleepier in the evenings and easier to put to bed. This meant my bedtime came at a more reasonable time too!

—*Michelle Davis-Dash, MD, a mom of a five-year-old son and a pediatrician, in Baltimore, MD*

                                         

When my daughter was around five years old, she developed sleep anxiety. She was afraid that someone was going to "come get her" in her sleep.

I filled a spray bottle with water and explained it was "monster spray." I let my daughter spray it each night before bed. This helped ease her mind.

I also talked with my daughter about what was bothering her. I encouraged her to write in a journal about it.

—*Eva Mayer, MD, a mom of a 12-year-old daughter and an 11-year-old son, an associate professor of pediatrics at Temple University, and a pediatrician with St. Luke's Hospital Coopersburg Pediatrics, in Pennsylvania*

When our daughter was five years old, she experienced sleep anxiety. It literally happened overnight, after I made a random comment that if she wanted to stay up late with her cousins, she would have to nap the next day. She hated napping and then started to worry that she wouldn't be able to fall asleep. The girl who slept for the most part through the night from eight weeks on suddenly wasn't able to get herself to sleep, and she was very anxious.

We tried to stay with our routine, but we ended up singing for 45 minutes or sitting by her bed and working on the laptop. This meant my husband and I could no longer visit in the evenings before bed as well.

After several months, we realized it still wasn't getting better. Then the anxiety about sleep began creeping into her daytime thoughts, so we found help. The first therapist we had a phone consult with wasn't helpful. We then had a few visits with a family and child therapist who specialized in anxiety, and that made a world of difference.

It's important to find help—the *right* help for your family—when sleep struggles are interrupting your life or causing worry for your child.

—*Katja Rowell, MD, a mom of a 10-year-old daughter, a family practice physician, and the author of* Helping Your Child with Extreme Picky Eating and Love Me, Feed Me *at TheFeedingDoctor.com, in St. Paul, MN*

## RALLIE'S TIP

*My youngest son was a mama's boy and a very opinionated child, and he did not want to go to preschool. Period.*

*Initially, it was a challenge to peel my son off me and leave him with his preschool teachers every day. My husband and I found that the best way to ease his anxiety and minimize his resistance was to casually walk into the classroom with him; get him interested in a toy, a classmate, or an activity; and then quietly drift away and out the door while his attention was directed elsewhere. This way, our son didn't have to watch us leave, which was really hard for him.*

*When we picked him up after school, we'd encourage him to tell us about his day, and we'd make a big deal about his artwork and papers.*

*Our son quickly realized that preschool was a fun and positive experience—and that he actually enjoyed it!*

### When to Call Your Doctor: Stress

It's often said that children are resilient, but that doesn't mean they don't sometimes need help to cope with a stressful life event, such as a death of someone close to them, divorce, a move, abuse, trauma, or an illness.

If a stressful event is affecting your child's sleep, or if it's causing behavior problems, moodiness, or changes in appetite, make an appointment with your doctor to discuss it. Your pediatrician might make a recommendation to see a child's therapist. A younger child who isn't old enough for school may need to see a doctor if she's showing delays in development.

## Sleep Walking and Sleep Talking

Sleep walking and sleep talking might be funny fodder for sit-coms and YouTube videos, but when it's your child sleep walking or sleep talking, it's not so funny. In fact, it can be downright scary.

∽◌∽

My older son sleepwalked one time. It was the scariest thing! Thankfully it happened only that one time when he was four years old. We have a home security system, and when he walked down the steps, the alarm went off and woke us up. We found him sound asleep in my husband's desk chair!

My younger son talks in his sleep—a lot! He has full conversations in his sleep to this day. My husband and I just ignore it.

—*Heather Orman-Lubell, MD, a mom of 15- and 11-year-old sons and a pediatrician in private practice at St. Chris Care at Yardley Pediatrics, in Pennsylvania*

∽◌∽

My younger daughter still sleepwalks and sleep talks, at eight years old. Her twin also sleepwalks. They each share a room with a sibling, and we try (their siblings more than us) to get them safely back to bed and keep them away from the stairs. We don't try to wake them.

Our son has washed several stuffed animals in the sink while sleepwalking and ended up alone in the kitchen searching for crayons. Our daughter can be fearful and upset when sleepwalking.

Our oldest used to get night terrors, and we would need to wake her. We would turn on the lights and try to wake her gently; otherwise, she would not stop screaming. It was the worst. She outgrew it by age four or so.

—*Rebecca Jeanmonod, MD, a mom of 12- and 8-year-old daughters and 11- and 8-year-old sons and a professor of emergency medicine and the associate residency program director for the emergency medicine residency at St. Luke's University Health Network, in Bethlehem, PA*

My boys didn't sleep walk, but I had a sleep walker sleep over at my house one night. It scared the daylights out of me!

—*Deborah Gilboa, MD, a mom of 14-, 12-, 10-, and 8-year-old sons, a family physician with Squirrel Hill Health Center, in Pittsburgh, PA, and a parenting speaker whose advice is found at AskDoctorG.com*

## Mommy MD Guides-Recommended Product
### *Indigo Dreams* and Indigo Dream Series

*Indigo Dreams* is a 60-minute relaxation audio book designed to entertain your child while introducing her to relaxation and stress management techniques. Four unique bedtime or naptime stories incorporate breathing, visualizations, progressive muscle relaxation, and affirmations. These are the same self-calming techniques recommended for adults but presented in a fun, interactive format that appeals to children. Children follow along with the characters as they learn diaphragmatic breathing with "A Boy and a Bear," make positive statements with "The Affirmation Web," visualize with "A Boy and a Turtle," and use progressive muscle relaxation with "The Goodnight Caterpillar." All four of these stories are also available as mp3 downloads, paperbacks, and eBooks.

*Indigo Dreams'* shorter stories are perfect for shorter attention spans and beginners. The story lengths range from 6 to 10 minutes. Each story introduces a different relaxation technique that children can use to relax, self-soothe, build self-esteem, and improve sleep. Female narration is accompanied by music, soothing sounds of crickets, gentle breezes, and forest animals. An additional 30-minute music sound track is included to further enhance your child's relaxation experience.

The Indigo Dreams Series includes Indigo Ocean Dreams, Indigo Dreams: Adult Relaxation, and Indigo Dreams: Kid's Relaxation Music. You can buy Indigo Dreams on **AMAZON.COM** for around $14.95 or downloads for $8.95. To experience the entire line of the Indigo Dreams Series visit **STRESSFREEKIDS.COM.**

## When to Call Your Doctor: Sleep Walking and Sleep Talking

Because sleep walking is relatively common among children, particularly kids between three and seven years old, and your child is likely to outgrow it in the coming years, there's no need to call the doctor in most cases.

The same goes for sleep talking. Talking, mumbling, and saying gibberish while asleep is usually short-lived and doesn't need treatment.

However, be aware that sleep walking happens more often among kids who have sleep apnea, and that is something that warrants a call to the pediatrician. If your little sleep walker also has symptoms of apnea, such as loud snoring and gasping for breath while sleeping, be sure to talk to your doctor about it.

## Combating Other Challenges

In 1964, a 17-year–old named Randy Gardner stayed awake for 11 days for a school science project. He holds the record for the longest anyone has gone without sleep.

Could you imagine being awake for 11 straight days? We can't either. Surely you're not dealing with anything so extreme! Hopefully that gives you a little comfort.

But still, whatever challenge you're facing is the biggest thing you have to contend with. And if your preschooler isn't sleeping well, you probably aren't either. Let's face it, you're only sleeping as well as your worst sleeping family member!

It might take some sleuthing to figure out what's keeping your preschooler awake, but you'll do it!

As a preschooler, my older son rarely slept. He had difficulty falling asleep and staying asleep. He wandered around our house at night. I tried everything: tough love, sticker charts, sitting with him, you name it. Finally, one day it clicked, and he started to sleep better at last. I think it was because he needed to grow into sleeping well.

—*Heather Orman-Lubell, MD*

❧

My son is ritualistic, and he has some rituals he has to do before he can go to sleep. He has to make sure that his closet door is closed tightly and make sure things are lined up just right on his dresser. It's not to the extent that it impacts his health or life; most of us have some compulsive behaviors.

We respect that about our son. We give him the space and time to do what he needs to do to settle down for sleep each night.

—*Lauren Hyman, MD, a mom of a 13-year-old daughter and an 11-year-old son and an ob-gyn at West Hills Hospital and Medical Center, in California*

❧

My boys sleep two to a room. Sometimes they stay up late talking and giggling or occasionally arguing. It's like having a sleepover every night—for good and for bad.

I think that this is very good relationship-building time for them. Even getting in trouble together is good for bonding. As long as my boys aren't being too loud or being mean to each other, I let them be. They often work things out on their own. I've never had to set any rules for talking, giggling, or arguing. If they're being loud, I simply go in and say, "That's it now. Go to sleep."

—*Deborah Gilboa, MD*

> **Control what you can control.**
> **Don't lose sleep worrying about things that you**
> **don't have control over because, at the end of the day,**
> **you still won't have any control over them.**
>
> —*Cam Newton, professional football player*

My son often wakes up before my husband and I do. He knows not to come wake us! Before bed, he puts a book right outside of his door. When he wakes up, he gets his book, crawls back into bed, and reads until it's time to get up.

—*Lauren Hyman, MD*

My boys enjoy having sleepovers with their friends. Sometimes it's hard for them to settle down and go to sleep. When that happens, I take a book and go sit on a chair in the room. Usually all I have to do is get them to be quiet for three minutes and at least one of the kids will fall asleep.

—*Deborah Gilboa, MD*

I think that it's important for parents to remember that there are times when things will throw sleep off for your kids, such as vacations, time changes, first days of school, and worries they might not share with you. It is important to be patient with them.

As an adult, I even have nights when I cannot sleep. It's important to help your children find tactics to handle those nights, which hopefully do not involve waking you up for every little thing they need or want.

My son had a good stretch of time when he could not fall asleep many nights while I was pregnant with our third baby. This was really challenging for all of us because I was tired and ready to deliver my baby. I really needed to sleep, and he was struggling with being unable to sleep nights when he wanted someone to just spend time with him. We had to work through ways to relax and read when he felt that way. In time he learned to be considerate of others' sleep schedules in the house.

—*Sigrid Payne DaVeiga, MD, a mom of 10-year-old and 1-month-old sons and a 5-year-old daughter and a pediatric allergist with the Children's Hospital of Philadelphia, in Pennsylvania*

∽⌀

I was fortunate that my kids didn't wake up a lot at night. When they were sick as toddlers or preschoolers and I was worried about them, I'd sleep next to them or we'd sleep together on the couch.

—*Kristy Magee, MD, a mom of 15-, 12-, and 8-year-old sons and a family physician at North Seminole Family Practice and Sports Medicine, in Sanford, FL*

## ? When to Call Your Doctor: Nightmares

Experts say up to half of all children age three to six have nightmares that are bothersome enough that they run or call to their parents. In most cases, a bedtime routine and relaxation before bed will help.

If nightmares are very disturbing to your child, you may want to call a psychologist who can use desensitization and relaxation therapies to reduce your child's anxiety.

# Chapter 25

## Sweet Dreams!

As you hold this book in your hands, you probably hold dozens of dreams in your head and wishes in your heart for your baby—and for yourself. What are those dreams?

Think of your dreams as if they were built out of tiny colorful LEGO blocks. You need to carefully put the pieces together to make your dreams come true. Certainly one of the pieces integral to accomplishing your dreams is getting enough sleep.

When you're sleeping, your body is focusing on your physical and mental well-being—literally preparing you for another busy day. After a good night of R and R—even one perchance to dream!—you hopefully awake feeling rested, rejuvenated, and ready to take on your next adventure!

### JUSTIFICATION FOR A CELEBRATION

When you find the courage to follow your dreams—celebrate!

> **"Dare to live the life you have dreamed for yourself. Go forward and make your dreams come true."**
> —*Ralph Waldo Emerson*

## Finding Hope for Older Kids

Your baby will sleep through the night. It might not be to-night, but it will be some-night. We promise. He will sleep through the night before he gets married, goes to college, in fact before he goes to kindergarten.

In 10 years or so, when your now-toddler is a teenager, and he wants to sleep til noon, you'll look back on this time of your life when you couldn't get him to sleep. Isn't parenting ironic?

My kiddos are 11 and 12, and they are *great* sleepers—at least for now. Who knows what will happen when they're teenagers! They never put up a fuss about getting up or going to bed.

My kids might be a little hesitant in the morning to get up, but they never give me a hard time. I think they also believe their little bodies work best with a routine, even on the weekends!

—*Antoinette Cheney, DO, a mom of a 12-year-old son and an 11-year-old daughter, and a family physician with Rocky Vista University College of Osteopathic Medicine, in Parker, CO*

### Take Time to Meditate

A parent's worries never end, especially when you have a new baby, and it can be hard to put those thoughts away when your head hits the pillow. But research has shown that using mindfulness meditation for 20 minutes a day can help you relax, which can lead to better sleep, according to Harvard Health Publications of the Harvard Medical School.

To meditate, focus on your breath, a short prayer, or a phrase and work on keeping your mind focused on the present rather than letting it wander. Download a free meditation app on your phone for soothing sounds to get you in a meditating mood.

My older kids are very good sleepers now. Everyone is in bed by 8:30 or 9 pm. I get them to bed and say good night. I need to have some *me* time too. From 4:30 pm each afternoon, I'm going nonstop between supervising my kids' homework, commuting to their activites, and running quick errands if needed. I like to have some time to myself to unwind from a loaded day at work and house duties. I usually lie in bed, reading a book or checking emails.

My oldest daughter can stay up a little bit to read, but by 10 pm she's usually falling asleep. My son falls asleep the minute his head hits the pillow. He's usually asleep by 9 pm. I'm so tired that I often fall asleep before my kids do.

*—Aline T. Tanios Keyrouz, MD, a mom of 13- and 7-year-old and 9-month-old daughters and an 11-year-son and an assistant professor of pediatrics at St. Louis University, in Missouri*

Today, at ages 12, 11, and 8, my kids still go to bed at 8 pm on weekdays and 8:30 pm on weekends. They typically all sleep together in one room on Friday and Saturday nights. They get up each morning at 7 am.

Their schedules remain pretty tightly regimented, but they do it entirely on their own now. I don't have to wake anyone for school or tell anyone it's time for bed. It's kind of nice!

*—Rebecca Jeanmonod, MD, a mom of 12- and 8-year-old daughters and 11- and 8-year-old sons and a professor of emergency medicine and the associate residency program director for the emergency medicine residency at St. Luke's University Health Network, in Bethlehem, PA*

Looking back, I remember that my daughters' early years really were the best of times and the hardest of times. On the one hand, it's joyful; it's meaningful. But on the other hand, you don't get many breaks, and you don't get your best rest during the early years. It was wonderful time, but simple things like taking a shower were an effort that took planning and organization.

*—Eva Ritvo, MD*

## Getting Sleep Yourself

Don't skimp on sleep. It's critical for your physical and mental health. You can actually live longer without food than you can without sleep.

Sleep deprivation affects your thinking and your emotions. You might feel loopy—even delirious. If you're sleep deprived, your immune system can't work properly. It might take you longer to recover from illness. Long-term sleep deprivation raises your risk of developing chronic illnesses, such as diabetes and heart disease.

The cure for all of these? Go to sleep!

I have found the most important thing that puts me in an okay state of mind for optimal functioning is sleep. If I've had a rough night, which often happens as an obstetrician, or worse yet a few bad nights, it's hard not to be cranky. I try my best to sleep well.

I consistently do a few things that help. I stop drinking caffeine at 2 pm. I exercise during the day, and I try to get yoga in a few times during the week, because I find they help me sleep better at night. I turn off all electronics a while before going to bed. I love to read in the evenings to settle down for the day. When I have the time, I meditate at night.

—*Lauren Hyman, MD, a mom of a 13-year-old daughter and an 11-year-old son and an ob-gyn at West Hills Hospital and Medical Center, in California*

When I look back at my daughters' baby and toddler years, I think, *Wow, that was a lot of work. I was tired a lot of the time.*

It's important for parents to be well rested. I tried to adapt my schedule, so I would go to bed early. Babies need a lot of sleep, and the best schedule for your baby might not be the best schedule for you. You need to align your baby's needs and yours so that everyone comes out ahead and gets some sleep.

—*Eva Ritvo, MD, a mom of two grown daughters, a psychiatrist, and a coauthor of* The Beauty Prescription, *in Miami Beach, FL*

Prioritizing sleep for baby *and mom* is important. I had a C-section, and I ended up with an infection. My baby and I had major breastfeeding struggles, so I was also pumping several hours a day.

But there was a benefit to bottlefeeding breast milk and formula: My husband and family members could enjoy feeding, and I could grab a little sleep—until my alarm went off to pump! Eventually, I stopped pumping. I felt guilty at the time, but looking back now, I wish I had stopped sooner.

Sleep deprivation and breastfeeding struggles increase the risk of postpartum depression and anxiety. Bonding with my baby and enjoying that time of life felt impossible while I was pumping on top of everything else.

—*Katja Rowell, MD, a mom of a 10-year-old daughter, a family practice physician, and the author of* Helping Your Child with Extreme Picky Eating and Love Me, Feed Me *at TheFeedingDoctor.com, in St. Paul, MN*

## RALLIE'S TIP

*When my children were babies, I was chronically sleep-deprived and exhausted. I didn't have trouble going to sleep, if I would only slow down long enough to shut my eyes.*

*Like most women, I found it difficult to give myself permission to rest. How could I sleep when there were dirty clothes piled knee-deep in the laundry room? Or when I couldn't find a single clean spoon in the kitchen?*

### How Much Sleep Do You Need?

Do we really need eight hours of sleep every night? The National Sleep Foundation and a panel of experts reviewed the literature about sleep and health. They concluded that adults ages 26 to 64 should get seven to nine hours of sleep a night. However, as few as six or as much as 10 hours of sleep may be appropriate. The experts didn't recommend going below or above the six to 10-hour range.

Eventually I accepted that I couldn't do everything. My babies were far more important to me than a having a spotless kitchen or being caught up on the laundry. I realized that I needed to be well rested to enjoy my children—and to be the kind of mother I wanted to be.

When I finally relaxed and gave myself permission to take a nap or go to bed when I was tired, everyone was happier. When your children are young, there will always be plenty of laundry and dirty dishes, but there are limited opportunities to rest, so sleep when you can—guilt free!

> **You're not healthy, unless your sleep is healthy.**
>
> **—William Dement, MD, PhD,**
> *the father of sleep medicine*

# Index

**Note:** <u>Underlined</u> references indicate boxed text.

# About the Authors

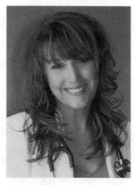

### RALLIE MCALLISTER, MD, MPH, MSEH

Dr. McAllister is a family physician and nationally known health expert. She is also a cofounder of Momosa Publishing LLC, publisher of MommyMDGuides.com and DaddyMDGuides.com and the Mommy MD Guides book series. She is a coauthor of *The Mommy MD Guide to Pregnancy and Birth, The Mommy MD Guide to Your Baby's First Year, The Mommy MD Guide to the Toddler Years,* and *The Mommy MD Guide to Losing Weight and Feeling Great.*

Dr. McAllister's nationally syndicated newspaper column, Your Health, appeared in more than 30 newspapers in the United States and Canada and was read by more than a million people each week.

A nationally recognized physician, Dr. McAllister has been the featured medical expert on more than 100 radio and television shows, including *Good Morning America Health, ABC News,* and *Fox News.* She's the former host of *Rallie on Health,* a weekly regional health magazine on WJHL News Channel 11 with more than one million viewers in a five-state area, and a weekly radio talk show. A dynamic public speaker, Dr. McAllister educates and entertains audiences from coast to coast with her upbeat, down-to-earth delivery of the latest health news.

Dr. McAllister is the author of several other books, including *Healthy Lunchbox: The Working Mom's Guide to Keeping You and Your Kids Trim,* and the founder of PonyUP! Kentucky, a company that creates unique, equestrian-style handbags and accessories to raise money to support rescued and retired horses. She is also a mother of three sons and a grandmother of three.

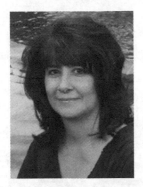

## Jennifer Bright Reich

Jennifer is a cofounder of Momosa Publishing LLC, publisher of MommyMD-Guides.com and DaddyMDGuides.com and the Mommy MD Guides book series. She is a coauthor of *The Mommy MD Guide to Pregnancy and Birth, The Mommy MD Guide to Your Baby's First Year, The Mommy MD Guide to the Toddler Years,* and *The Mommy MD Guide to Losing Weight and Feeling Great.*

Jennifer is a writer and editor with more than 15 years of publishing experience. She has contributed to more than 150 books and published more than 100 magazine and newspaper articles.

Jennifer's credits include writing *The Babyproofing Bible* (Fair Winds, 2007), contributing writing to 12 books in the *How to Survive Guide* book series, including *How to Survive Your Baby's First Year* (Hundreds of Heads, 2004), project editing the *New York Times* bestsellers *The South Beach Diet Cookbook* (Rodale, 2004) and *The South Beach Diet Good Fats/Good Carbs Guide* (Rodale, 2004), copyediting *Kitty Bartholomew's Decorating ABCs* (Rodale, 2005), cowriting *The Outwit Your Weight Journal* (Rodale, 2002), and writing more than a dozen articles for *Prevention* magazine, as well as articles for various newspapers.

Jennifer honed her planning and organizing skills during four years in the Reserve Officer Training Corps at the University of Pennsylvania and while serving for four years as a lieutenant in the U.S. Army, including one year working directly for the three Commanding Generals of I Corps at Fort Lewis, WA.

After that, Jennifer worked for seven years on staff at Rodale before launching her own editorial services business, Bright Communications LLC, in 2004.

Jennifer lives near Allentown, PA, with her two sons.

# ALSO BY
# MOMOSA PUBLISHING LLC

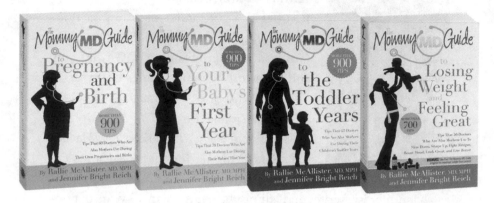

• Order our books online at many sites, including
Walmart.com, Amazon.com, and MommyMDGuides.com

• Purchase them at bookstores nationwide

• Download them for your Kindle, Nook, or iPhone/iPad

Enjoy more Mommy MD Guides' tips on

The Mommy MD Guide to Pregnancy and Birth app.

Visit us at MommyMDGuides.com

and DaddyMDGuides.com.

## COMING SOON!

*The Mommy MD Guides are hard at work on more titles in the series.
Keep a lookout for:*

*The Mommy MD Guide to Surviving Morning Sickness*

*The Mommy MD Guide to the School Years*